MIND DIET

Eating for a
Sharp Mind and
Healthy Brain

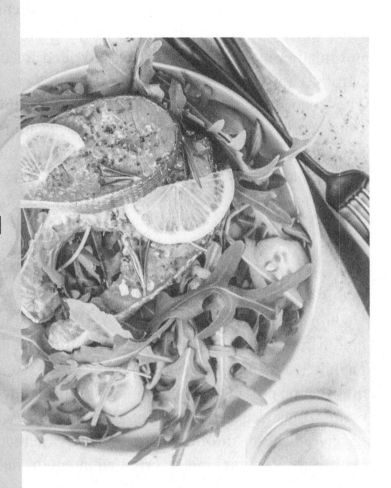

Garry Goodman

LEGAL & DISCLAIMER

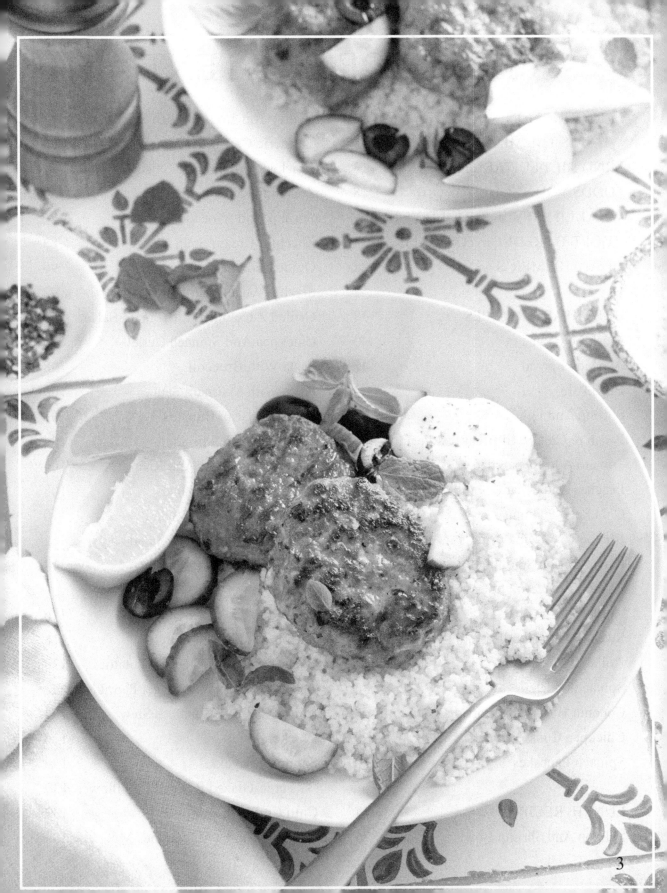

TABLE OF CONTENT

INTRODUCTION 6

WHAT IS THE MIND DIET 8

MIND DIET SUITABLE FOODS 13

FOODS YOU SHOULD AVOID 18

WHAT LIFESTYLE SHOULD YOU
ADOPT TO REDUCE YOUR RISK
OF ALZHEIMER'S 22

BREAKFAST RECIPES 38

Mushroom Omelet 40

Avocado Spread 42

Bean Pate 44

Shrimp And Eggs Mix 46

Peach & Chia Seed Breakfast Parfait 48

Tomato And Eggs Salad 50

Peaches And Cream 52

Chia Seed Pudding 54

Blueberry & Mint Parfaits 56

Kiwi Spinach Smoothie 58

Raspberry Overnight Oats 60

Apple Oats 62

Sweet Potato Noodles With
Hollandaise Sauce 64

Spinach Omelet 66

Coconut Buckwheat Porridge 68

Chickpea Cookie Dough 70

Spinach Pancakes 72

LUNCH RECIPES 74

Salmon And Shrimp Bowls 76

Cherry Tomato And Corn Salad 78

Turmeric Carrot Cream 80

Chicken And Spinach Salad 82

Zucchini Cakes 84

Shrimp And Avocado Mix 86

Zucchini Cream Soup 88

Quinoa Edamame Salad 90

Sizzling Vegetarian Fajitas 92

Grilled Zucchini With Tomato Salsa 94

Chickpea And Spinach Cutlets 96

Pasta With Broccoli 98

Pasta With Marinara Sauce 100

Rice And Bean Burritos 102

Air Fryer Pumpkin Slices 104

Smoky Red Beans And Rice 106

Coriander Shrimp Salad 108

Turkey And Endives Salad 110

Shrimp And Asparagus Salad 112

Spice-Roasted Carrots 114

DINNER RECIPES 116

Shrimp And Zucchini Pan 118

Black Bean Stuffed Sweet Potatoes 120

Baked Chicken With Sweet Paprika 122

Chickpeas And Tomatoes Stew 124

Chicken Pieces 126

Salmon Teriyaki 128

Balsamic-Glazed Roasted Cauliflower 130

Chili Cod 132

Chicken Thighs And Grapes Mix 134

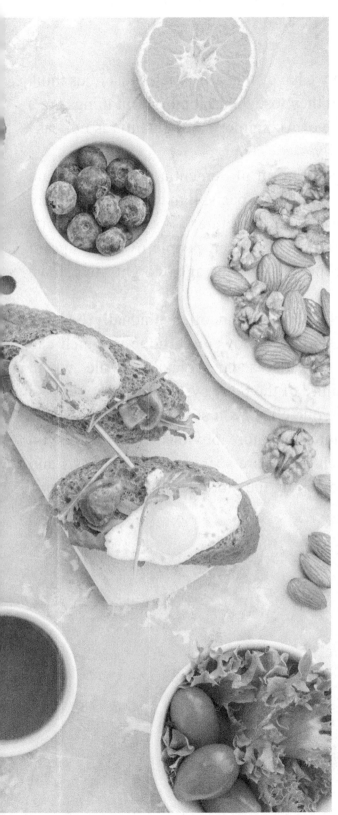

Coconut Chickpea Curry   136

Cauliflower And Tomatoes Mix   138

Cauliflower Steak With Sweet-Pea Puree   140

Ginger Sesame Halibut   142

Bolognese Pasta   144

Thyme Chicken Mix   146

Tasty Roast Salmon   148

Linguine With Wild Mushrooms   150

Spaghetti With Chickpeas Meatballs   152

Cashew Turkey Medley   154

DESSERTS & SNACKS   156

Cucumber Salad   158

Baked Carrot Chips   160

Peanut Butter Popcorn   162

Zucchini Dip   164

Carrot Cashew Pate   166

Apples And Yogurt   168

Cauliflower Popcorn   170

Rainbow Fruit Salad   172

Marinated Olives   174

Simple Banana Cookies   176

Cranberry Squares   178

Cookie Dough Bites   180

Potato Chips   182

Lentils Spread   184

Roasted Walnuts   186

CONCLUSION   188

INTRODUCTION

Alzheimer's disease is something that we have all heard about. Most of us think it occurs only in older people, and that they lose their memory. But things are a little bit different. Facing the diagnose of Alzheimer's or dementia is not easy for the patient, let alone for their family.

Alzheimer's disease is the most common form of dementia, which is a brain disorder that impacts the person's living on daily basis. It manifests in the form of memory loss and cognitive changes. The Alzheimer's Association reports that not all memory loss is Alzheimer's. One in ten people over the age of sixty-five, and almost one-third of the people over the age of eighty-five, have Alzheimer's.

The symptoms of this disease slowly develop and often gradually become worse as time goes by. Things may start with slow forgetfulness, which can widespread brain impairment. This happens as the critical cells die, which causes drastic personality loss and failure of the body system.

You cannot diagnose Alzheimer's by yourself. If you suspect that you or your loved one have it (signs become more and more obvious), make sure you schedule a doctor's appointment. Even if you are scared, early diagnosis and help will give you a better chance of delaying the more debilitating symptoms.

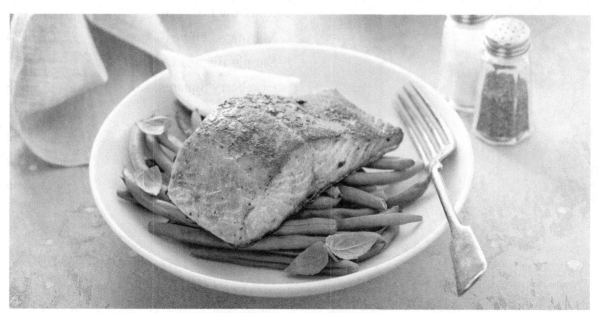

With suitable medicine, you are prolonging your independent and make the most of your life.

And although Alzheimer's disease is common and older people aren't immune to it, there are things you can do to prevent it. The first thing is changing your diet and lifestyle.

Many people aren't aware that the food they eat and the way they live their lives affect their health in the long run (even if they are perfectly healthy in the present moment).

This book is written specially to help you learn the benefits of the MIND diet. Every chapter carefully selects important things such development, and diagnosing of Alzheimer's, suitable foods that the MIND diet recommends, and changes in lifestyle that should help you lower the risk of developing this disease.

This books' premise is to help you learn how to prevent Alzheimer's disease and dementia by changing your eating habits and your lifestyle. Information is crucial in any segment of life. The earlier you get the needed info, the faster you can start taking action and prevent larger damage.

It is never too early to change your life and develop good habits that may later save your life and allow you to live your older years in peace.

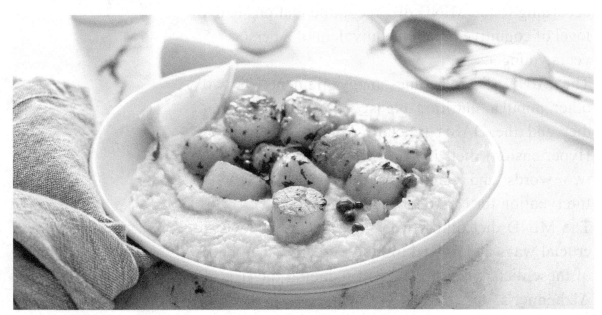

WHAT IS THE MIND DIET

You have probably heard that saying, "you are what you eat." These are words of wisdom, and even your doctor will confirm that. The food you consume abundantly affects your brain and its functions.

According to a new study done by Rush University Medical Center in Chicago, there is a way to reduce the risk of Alzheimer's disease by an actual diet. They called it the MIND diet, and the breathtaking results are that this diet reduces the risk for as much as 53 percent. Even if a person doesn't strictly follow the MIND diet, they can be in quite a good shape and reduce the risk of this disease by one third.

The study was published in the journal Alzheimer's & Dementia, checked at more than nine hundredth people between the ages of fifty-eight and ninety-eight who filled out food questionnaires and had several repeated neurological testing. The results showed that the participants whose diets were according to the MIND diet recommendations had a level of cognitive function equivalent of a person 7.5 years younger.

The MIND diet combines many elements of two other popular nutrition plans – the Mediterranean diet and the DASH (Dietary Approaches to Stop Hypertension) diet. In fact, MIND is a mix of the two words and stands for Mediterranean-DASH Intervention for Neurodegenerative Delay.)

The MIND diet differs from those plans in several crucial ways and proved to more effective than both of these diets when it comes to reducing the risk of Alzheimer's.

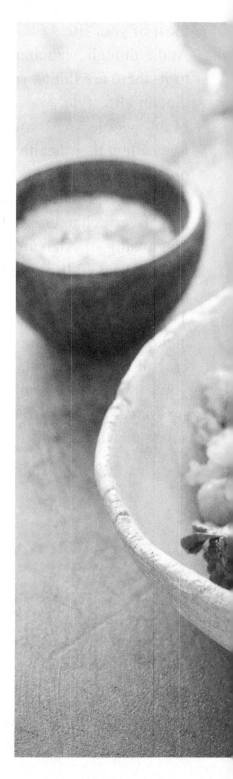

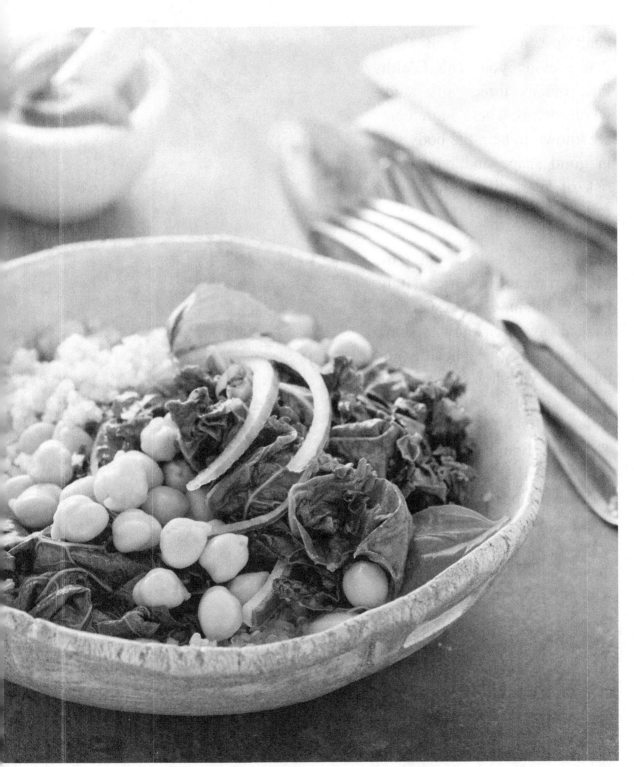

Now, let's focus briefly on the Mediterranean diet. It is considered to be one of the healthiest diets rich in foods that provide you with healthy fats, omega three fatty acids, whole grains. These ingredients are known to help the body stay in good shape and reduce the risk of heart disease and some cancers.

People who live in the Mediterranean countries (Italy, France, Spain, Greece, Croatia) have always been known to have slender figures, lead healthy and long lives with low risks of heart issues, and other evil diseases.

The thing about this diet is that it is focused on eating whole foods. There is no place for processed foods in this diet. Fruits, vegetables, olive oil, fish, nuts, the moderate consummation of wine are just a few of the things this diet offers. When you cleanse your body of sugars, unhealthy fats, and junk food, you aren't exposing yourself to the risk of high cholesterol, heart failures, or other diseases.

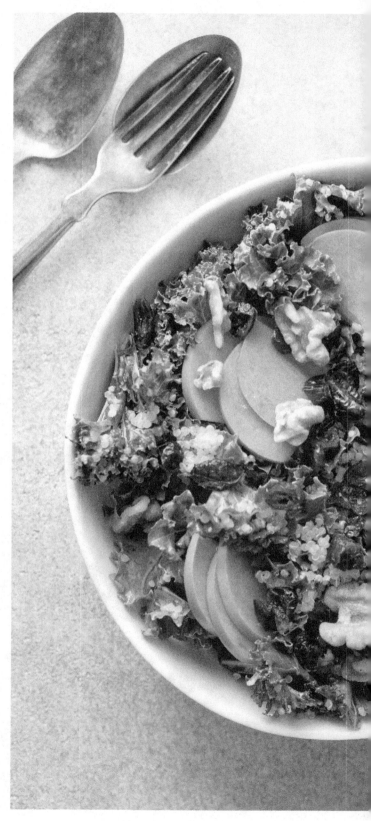

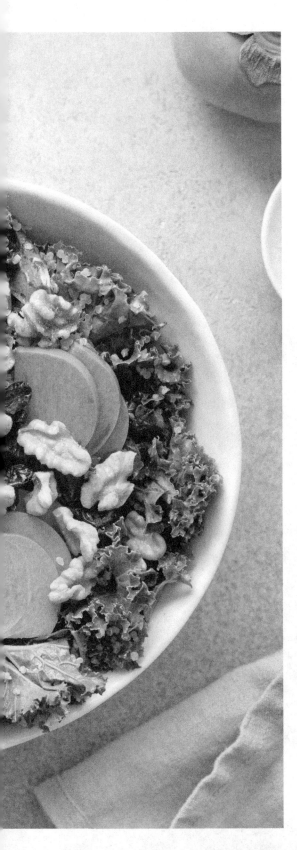

The DASH diet is focused on fruits and vegetables and low-fat dairy and is especially beneficial if you want to reduce the risk of stroke, heart attack, or hypertension.

Boosting your diet with flavonoid-rich produce may benefit the mind. According to a study published in Annals of Neurology, fruits like strawberries, blueberries, or strawberries are known to prevent cognitive aging in women by up to two and a half years.

There is a link between eating leafy green vegetables (kale, spinach) and reduced inflammation and oxidative stress (these two are associated with Alzheimer's disease, according to a study published in the Journal of the Academy of Nutrition and Dietetics. In general, food that is rich in antioxidants and can help lower inflammation and oxidative stress.

Oxidative stress happens when antioxidant defences are low, and the body can't fight toxic molecules (free radicals). This stress causes cell damage in the brain and the body, and it has been connected with several diseases, including cancer and Alzheimer's.

The MIND diet is mainly focused on consuming plant-based foods and reducing the intake of animal products and foods high in saturated fat. So, what exactly do you need to eat to have a proper MIND diet? In the next chapter, we will focus on the foods that are suitable for this diet.

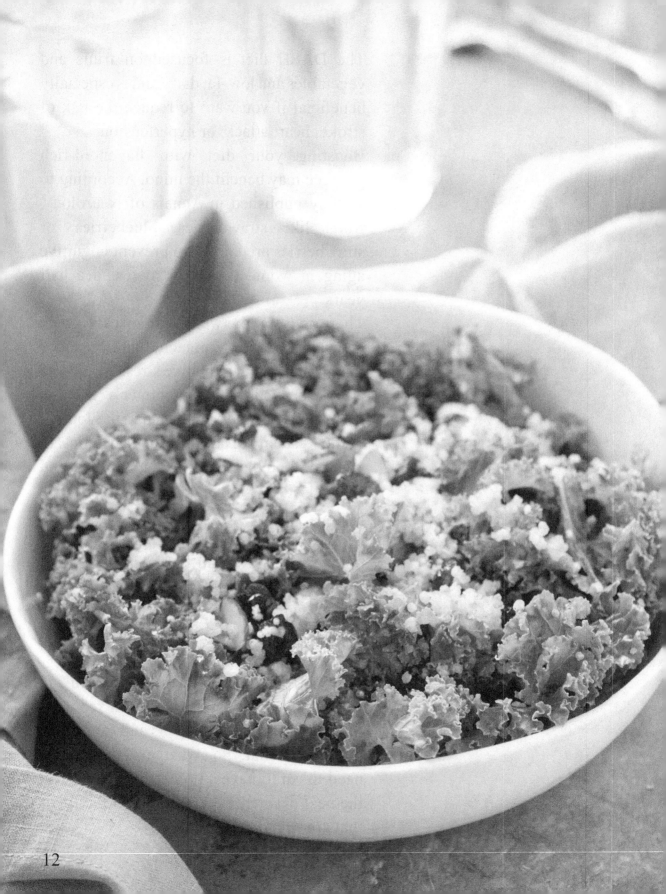

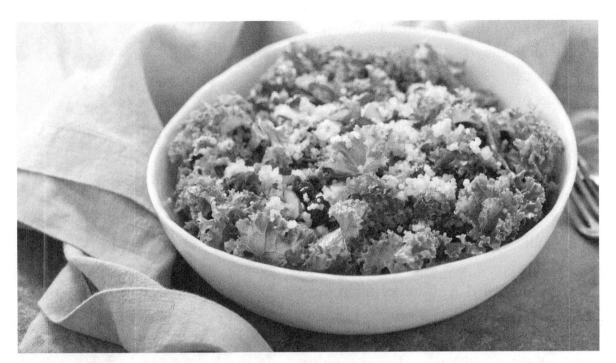

MIND DIET SUITABLE FOODS

Most people think that a diet is only meant to help you lose weight or detox your body. But, not every diet is supposed to help you lose weight. Various diets provide various results. The MIND diet, as mentioned in the previous chapters, is meant to help you improve you're your brain health and keep Alzheimer's disease at bay.

As I already mentioned in the previous chapter, this diet is not supposed to be followed by people who fear that they might be at risk of getting Alzheimer's, but by anyone who wants to keep their brain in good shape for as long as possible.

You don't have to be an older person to start this diet. You can be in your twenties, thirties, or forties and start consuming fresh fruits and vegetables, reduce the amount (or completely stop consuming) processed and junk food, eat healthy fats, seafood, and lower amounts of sugar, processed meat, and unhealthy fats.

Here are the foods that are suitable for this diet. I want to point out that you do not have to have weight issues to start this diet.

The MIND diet is all about fresh vegetables. The first thing that you should incorporate in your menu is more frequent servings of leafy green vegetables such as spinach, kale, but also collards, broccoli, and other green vegetables. They are packed in vitamin A and C, iron, and other nutrients. If you are not used on eating lots of vegetables, please start with small steps. Include a bowl of salad at least twice a week (although salads are recommended with every main meal of the day). Besides a salad, you can consume broccoli in the form of steamed side vegetables with your dinner (poultry or past, for example).

According to researchers, six or more servings of green vegetables per week will give you the best benefits. I would like to point out that DASH and the Mediterranean diet do not specifically recommend the upper mentioned vegetables, but the MIND diet study shows that these leafy green vegetables make a difference with the risk of getting Alzheimer's.

The MIND diet is focused on the importance of vegetables for your brain health. According to researchers, it is recommendable to consume a salad and at least one vegetable every day. It is the only way to reduce the risk of getting Alzheimer's.

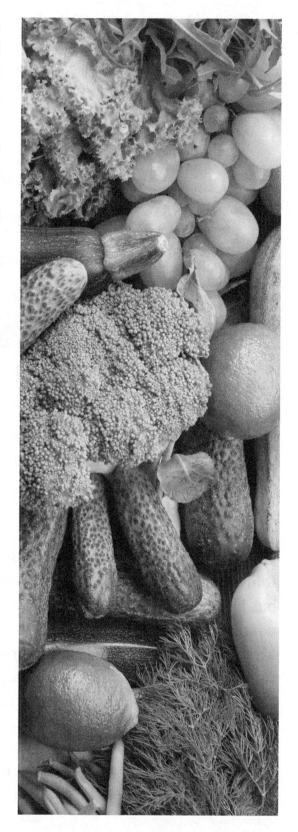

Next on the list of the MIND diet, suitable foods are nuts. They are lovely and healthy snacks. Nuts are rich in healthy fats, antioxidants, fiber, and will keep you full in between meals. Studies have shown that nuts help in lowering bad cholesterol and reduce the risk of heart diseases. If you are going to follow the MIND diet, you should eat nuts at least five times a week.

When it comes to fruits, berries are the only fruit that is especially recommended in this diet. All berries are great, but blueberries are one of the most potent foods that protect the brains' health. Strawberries are also excellent and provide good brain health and cognitive function. You should consume berries at least twice a week. It is an excellent extra for your breakfasts and healthy snacks.

Next on this list are beans. If you don't have the habit of consuming beans, now it is the perfect time to start. Beans are known for their high amount of proteins and fiber (excellent food for vegans and vegetarians as well) and are low in fat and calories. They will keep your mind sharp, and the MIND diet includes them in its menu. According to researches, beans should be on your menu at least three times a week.

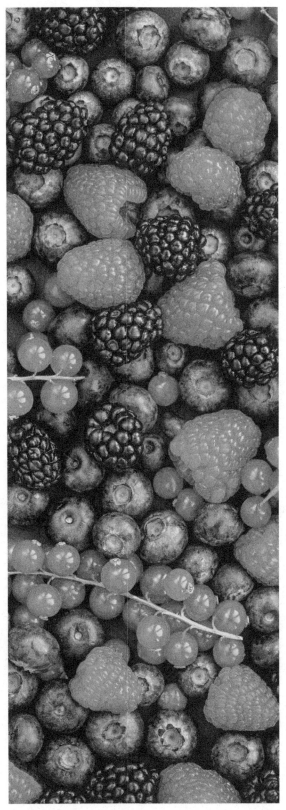

You don't have to be a doctor or a nutritionist to know that whole grains are especially important in any healthy diet. At least three servings a day is the MIND diet recommendation.

If you worried that there is no meat in this diet, here it is. According to this diet, you should consume fish at least once per week. Fish protects brain function, but it should not be consumed too frequently. Compared to the Mediterranean diet (which recommends consuming fish almost every day), the MIND diet limits it to once a week.

Poultry is also recommended to keep your brain healthy in the long run. The MIND diet recommends two or more servings per week.

Cooking is essential for any diet if you want to be sure that all your meals will be properly prepared. Olive oil is known for its healthy fats and is recommended to be used for cooking. According to researchers, people who used olive oil as their main oil had bigger protection of their cognitive decline.

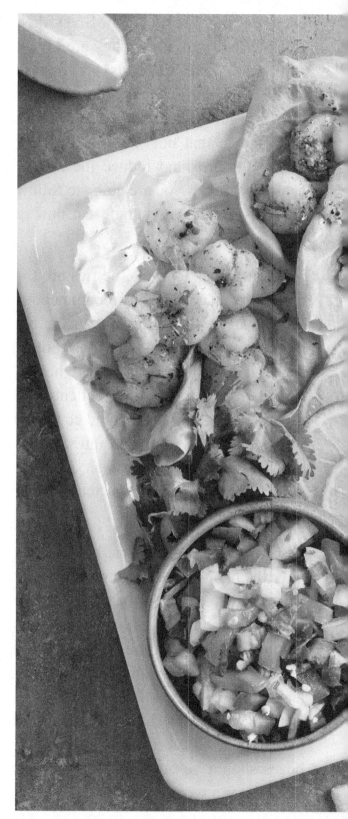

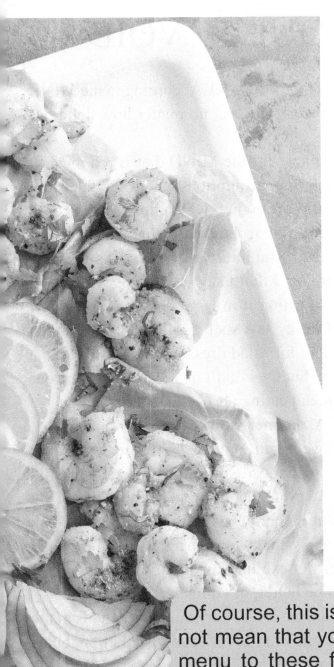

This diet, as well, allows you to drink wine. You can drink one glass of wine every day (not more than one, though). So, make sure to celebrate and raise a toast of the fantastic MIND diet that is protecting your brain in the long run.

If any of these foods are not suitable for you for any reason (you're a vegan or vegetarian, allergic to any of these foods), don't quit the MIND diet. Researches show that the MIND diet can be followed moderately and that even in that case, it reduces the risk of Alzheimer's disease.

Of course, this is a just a shortlist, and it does not mean that you should reduce your weekly menu to these foods only. You can combine them with other foods such as pasta, healthy desserts, Greek yogurt, and so on. The more you include leafy greens, berries, fish, and olive oil in your diet, the better.

FOODS YOU SHOULD AVOID

Every diet recommends foods to eat and foods to avoid. According to the MIND diet, there are specific foods that don't work for you, no matter how delicious they are.

The first one on the list of foods not suitable for the MIND diet is red meat. It is not forbidden, but it should be limited to consumption to no more than four times per week. Compared to the Mediterranean diet, which limits red meat to once a week, that is far better (if you are a fan of red meant, that is).

When it comes to unhealthy fats, make sure you limit your intake of butter and margarine to less than a tablespoon per day. I don't say it will be easy for you to quit it, especially if you were used to eating it in large amounts every day, but stay patient. Keep your focus on healthy fats such as olive oil; it is much healthier and much better for cooking and for salad dressings.

Milk products such as cheese taste great, but they don't do a good favor to your brain. The MIND diet does not recommend eating cheese for more than once a week if you want to reduce the risk of Alzheimer's.

You already know that pastries and sweets, in general, aren't really health, although we can agree that they taste delicious. Consuming sweets on daily basis is not the best choice if you want to protect your brain health. The MIND diet is not excluding sweets entirely but recommends a limit of no more than five of your favorite sweet treats per week. Which, you can agree, is quite a good thing. Unlike other diets, this one does not exclude sugar entirely, although if you can consume more fruits, it would be better, of course.

Fast food and fried foods, in general, is on the list of very unhealthy foods in the MIND diet. Yes, it tastes great, and it creates a mild (or severe) addiction, but if you are going to follow this diet, then you will have to reduce the consumption of junk food to once a week only. Not only will it help you keep your weight balanced, but it will also help you maintain your brain health and your general health as well. Researchers say that limiting your consumption of these foods is solely because they contain saturated fats and trans fats. Studies show that trans fats are closely connected with various diseases, including Alzheimer's disease.

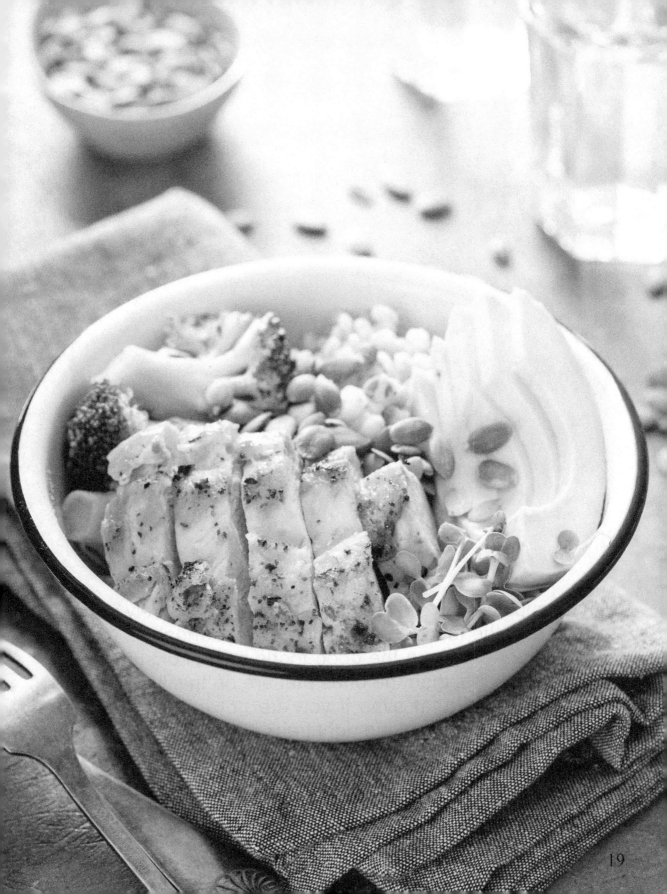

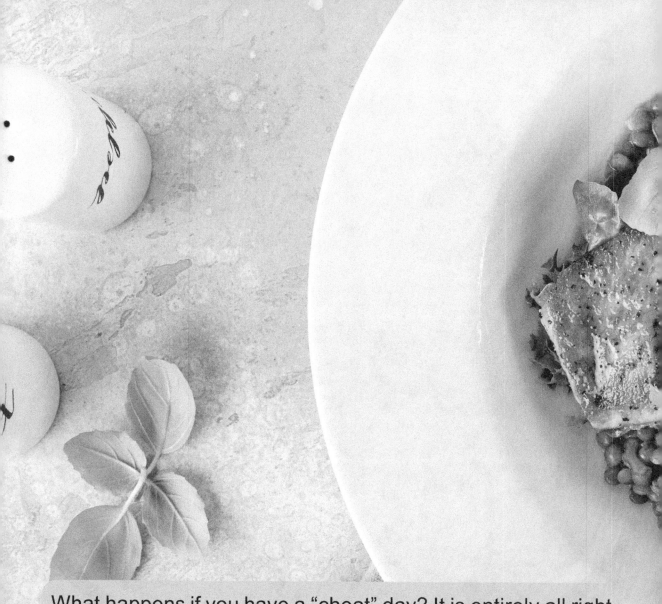

What happens if you have a "cheat" day? It is entirely all right to reach for the foods that are not recommendable. You will still have benefits from the good foods if you consume them in larger amounts than the ones that are on this list.

Researchers say that even if you are not following entirely this diet, you are still on the right track of reducing the risk for Alzheimer's disease. All you need to do is stick with this diet for a long time and get enough protection, a healthy functioning body, and good health.

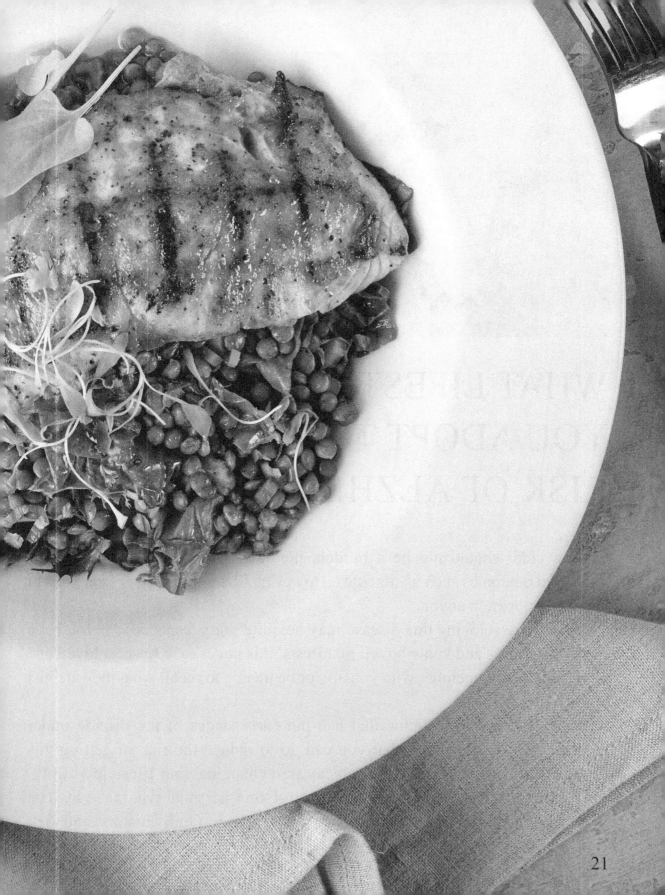

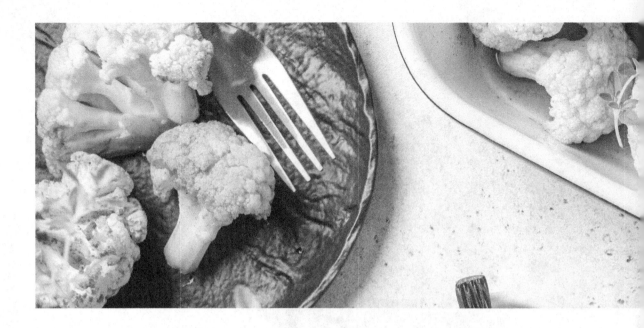

WHAT LIFESTYLE SHOULD YOU ADOPT TO REDUCE YOUR RISK OF ALZHEIMER'S

Getting older should not be a burden, nor it should bring you the fear of unwanted outcomes such as illnesses. However, Alzheimer's disease is present and may happen to anyone.

The idea of developing this disease may be quite scary, especially if you have faced this illness and know how it manifests. It is never easy to see a loved one being unable to remember who you are, or be unable to recall what they ate just a few minutes before.

Although there is a medicine that can put early stages of the disease under control, there is something that you can do to reduce the risk of getting this disease. Besides the MIND diet, you can start changing your lifestyle as well.

First of all, make sure to identify and control your personal risk that may lead to potential risk. It can be anything such as age, genes, family history, and diet.

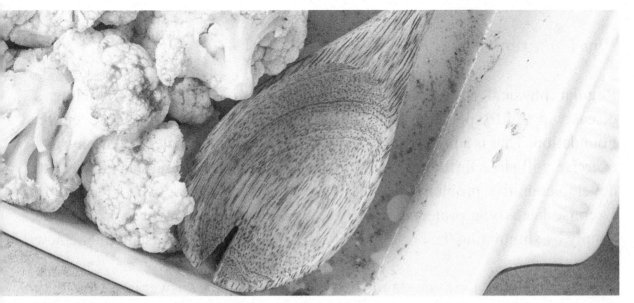

Once you do that, you will know how you can maximize your chances of a healthy brain for as long as you live. These steps will help you keep Alzheimer's disease at bay and will slow the process of deterioration.

As I mentioned, Alzheimer's is a complex disease, and there are several factors. Some of these factors are your age and genetics, and you truly cannot do much about them. But, there are seven other pillars that you can control, which can help you keep your brain in a healthy state. Here they are:

- Regular exercise
- Healthy diet
- Social engagement
- Mental stimulation
- Quality sleep
- Stress management
- Vascular health

Although, in the past, doctors believed that this disease is mainly linked with age, today, experts believe that Alzheimer's cannot be limited to age only. In fact, brain issues may start a long time before they are identified, even in the middle age. That means that you are never too old to start taking care of your brain health. The more you keep the upper mentioned pillars strong, the longer they will serve you and will offer you stronger support.

Let's see each of these seven bullet points in detail.

Physical exercise

Regular physical activity will reduce the risk of developing Alzheimer's disease up to fifty percent, according to Alzheimer's Research & Prevention Foundation. That is a big amount, you will agree. Besides that, regular physical exercise will slow further deterioration in people who have already started to develop cognitive problems.

Exercise keeps you protected from Alzheimer's and other types of dementia simply by stimulating the brain's ability to keep old connections and make new ones.

If you wonder how long you should exercise per week, the answer is not less than 150 minutes per week. The best combination is cardio and strength exercises. If you are new to physical exercise, start with something that you can do easily, such as walking or swimming.

Start with moderate levels of weight and resistance training to increase muscle mass, but also to keep your brain health. If you are older than sixty-five, add two to three strength sessions in your weekly exercising routine.

Next, you should include coordination and balance exercises. Head injuries that happen because of falling increase the risk of getting Alzheimer's disease or dementia. Keeping your head protected is essential, and it can happen if you can maintain good balance and coordination. Make sure you always wear a helmet when you cycle or do some other risky physical activity. The best balance and coordination exercises are Tai Chi, yoga, and Pilates (use balance balls).

If you were not active so far, the beginning may be challenging for you. You may feel that you cannot do anything, or that things seem difficult. Keep in mind that a little workout is better than nothing. So, start with baby steps. You may not be ready for the gym, but you can always walk around the block, use the stairs, or go for a swim. All it takes is a ten-minute walk per day to begin your physical exercise. Then gradually build your physical activity to half an hour per day, then maybe start hiking, swimming, or doing light yoga.

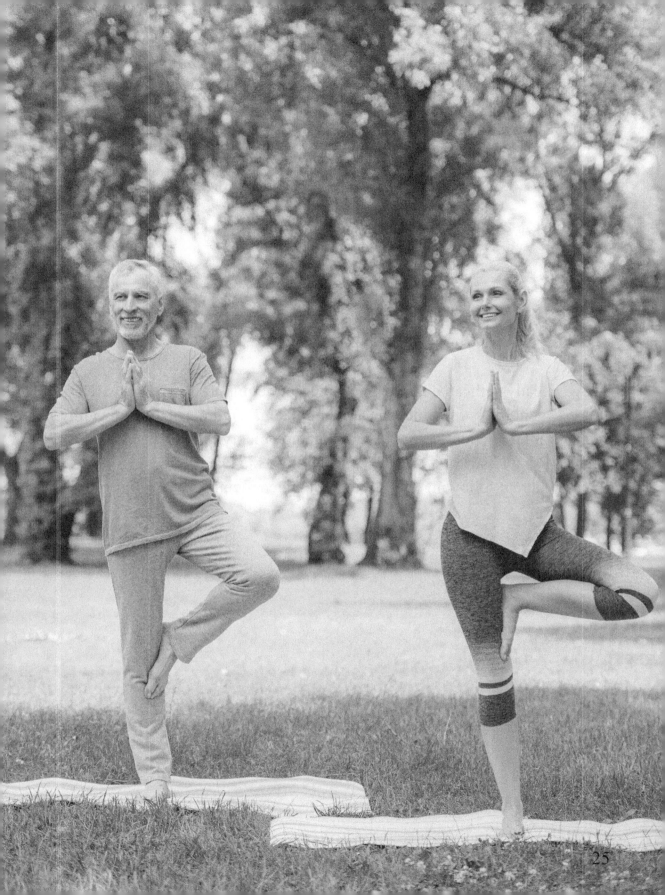

Healthy Diet

I have already dedicated an entire chapter to the importance of the MIND Diet. It is essential that you reduce the amount of sugar, red meat, and unhealthy fats such as butter and margarine. Instead, include plenty of leafy green vegetables, berries, fish and seafood once a week, poultry, nuts, and olive oil.
Even moderate following the MIND diet is beneficial for your brain.

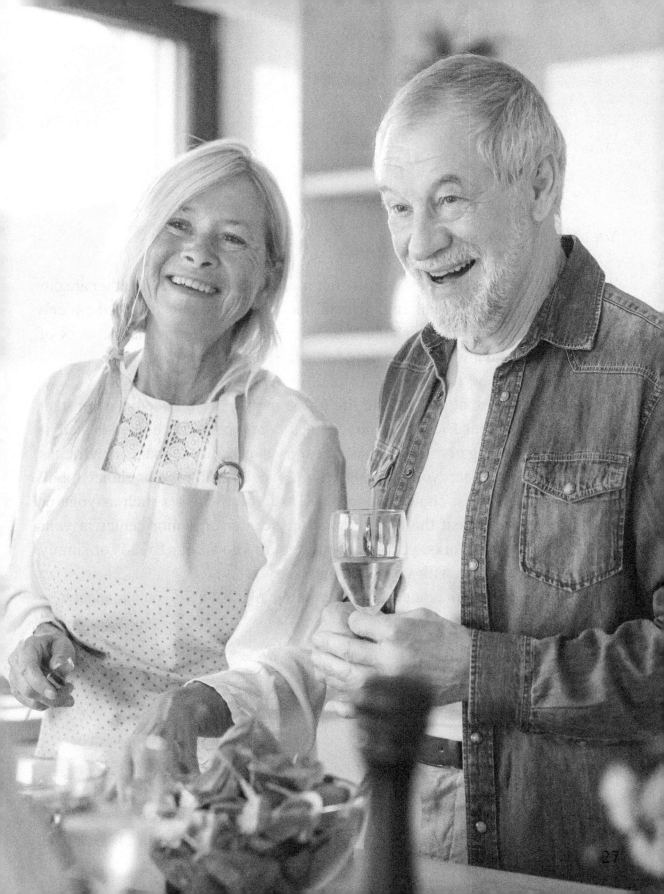

Social Engagement

We are highly social creatures who are not made for isolation, and neither are our brains. Keeping your social engagement may protect you against Alzheimer's disease and dementia in your older age, so make build your social network of friends steady and always make time for some social interaction.

It is not necessary that you are the life of the party. All you need is a constant connection with your friends and loved ones. Many people become isolated as they age, but making new friends has no expiry date. You can make new friends at any age. You can start volunteering or join a social club of your choice (book club, support sessions, choir, and so on). Take group classes such as yoga or Pilates, or you can visit the local community center or senior center in your area. If none of this works, you can always get to know your friends or simply schedule weekly dates with your old friends.

Go to the museum, park, concerts, or any public place where you can meet new people and simply talk to them.

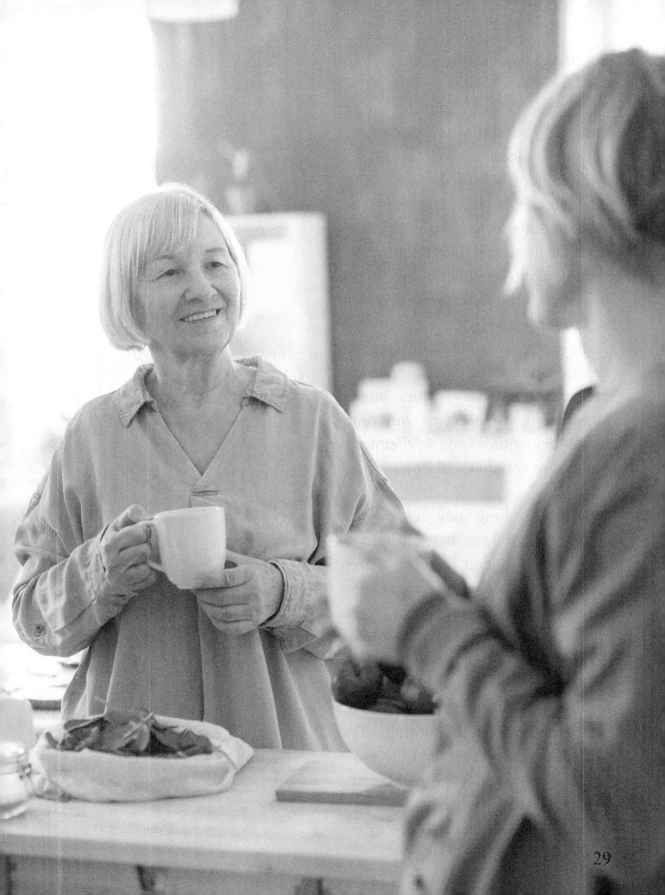

Mental Stimulation

The process of learning never ends. If you stimulate your mental activity by learning new things, you will reduce the risk of developing Alzheimer's disease and dementia. Older adults who spend about ten sessions of mental training improved their cognitive functioning. They also show long-lasting improvement in further years.

Activities such as interaction, organization, and communication are excellent ways for mental stimulation. To prevent your brain from dementia and Alzheimer's, make sure you do the following.

Learn something new every day – Schedule at least half an hour of your day to spend learning a new thing such as a foreign language, or practise a musical instrument. If this seems like something you cannot do (because of various reasons), practice something new. Perhaps us a different road to get home, or get a new hobby such as knitting. The greater the new thing, and the more complex and challenging it is, the better the benefit.

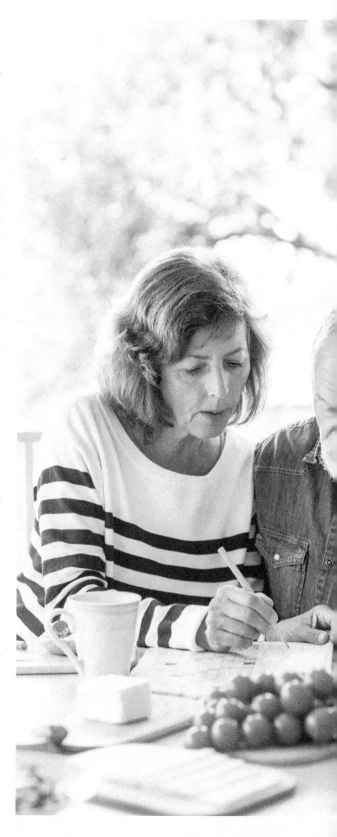

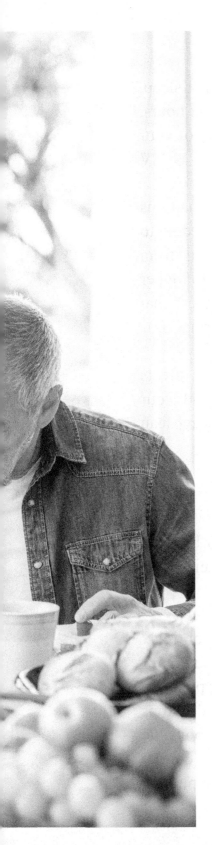

Challenge yourself with an existing activity - If you're not fond of learning something new every day, you can still challenge your brain by challenging your skills and knowledge of something you are familiar with. Let's say you know how to play the piano and don't want to learn a new instrument; then, commit to learn a new piece of music every day or improve the piece you already know how to play.

Practice memorization – There are many games that can help you achieve this. For example, you can create a sentence in which every first word starts with the letter of the initial of your dear person. Let's say you have friends with the following names Harry, Lola, Iris, Tony; create a sentence that says, "How Lovely Is Today." Such a memorization technique will keep your brain busy, and you will surely create some nice mantras for the day.

Play strategy games, riddles, and puzzles - Brain teasers and strategy games are great mental exercise. These games will help you build your capacity to create and retain cognitive associations. You can always get a crossword puzzle, play cards or board games, Scrabble or Sudoku.

Go to the less traveled road - We are all creature of habits that tend to create zone of comforts. But, make sure to stimulate your brain by using the less traveled road. Not only you will see new things, but it will surely be a great brain exercise. Also, try to use your less dominant hand more.

Get Some Sleep

Our bodies are not meant to go through life without proper sleep. With age, people tend to get enough sleep after five or six hours. But, it is essential that you should never ruin the quality of your sleep by ruining your rest schedule, use phone, laptop, or TV before bed or read or listen to stressful news.

There are many links between lack of sleep or poor sleep patterns and the development of Alzheimer's and dementia. According to some studies, quality sleep is essential for flushing out toxins from the brain. There are studies that have linked poor sleep to higher levels of beta-amyloid in the brain (this is a sticky protein that can disrupt the deep sleep that is crucial for memory formation).

If you were ever sleep deprived, you already know how it affects your thinking and cognitive activities. It affects your mood, your physical movements, and you react slower. Lack of sleep can highly affect the development of Alzheimer's disease.

Here is what you can do to improve your sleep:

Set a regular sleep schedule – It is important to go to bed and wake up at the same time. It reinforces your natural circadian rhythms. Your brain's clock loves regularity.

Set the mood for a sleep – Your bed is a place where you relax and sleep. It should not be a place for television, computers, or phones. Although it is very challenging, don't take your phone in bed with you. The blue light is messing up your brain, and it stops it from producing melatonin, which is a hormone responsible for sleep. Make sure your room is darkened, with the correct temperature and that your mattress is cozy and does not put any pressure on your body.

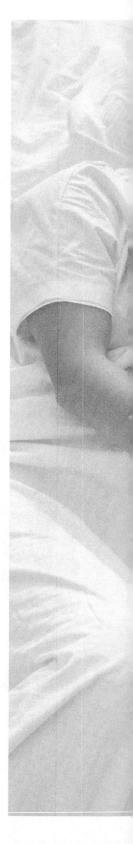

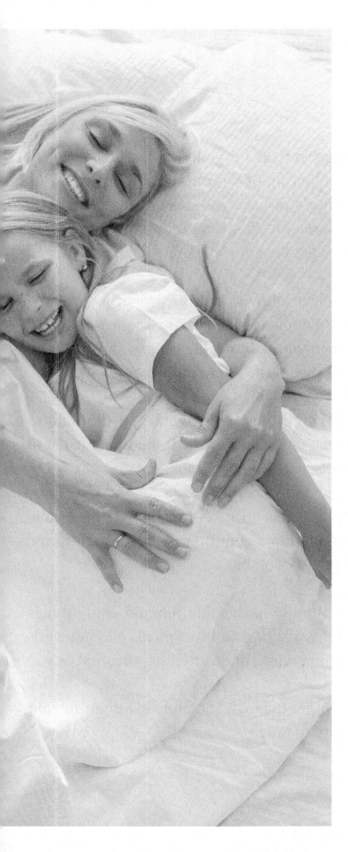

You can make a relaxing bedtime ritual – Do some light stretches before bed, or take a hot bath. Your body should relax before you fall asleep. You can also listen to relaxing music or meditate in a darkened room. Once you make this a habit, it would feel natural to do it, and your brain will link these activities with your sleep time.

Quiet your mind – Although quieting the mind can be quite a challenge, it is not impossible. Regular meditations can help you reduce your anxiety, negative self-talk, and worrying. Give yourself at least fifteen to thirty minutes of meditation before bed (make sure nobody disturbs you and that all the sounds on your phone are off).

Check if you have sleep apnea – People who snore often have sleep apnea. If this is the case with you, schedule a screening. Sleep apnea means that you don't breathe properly and that there are precious seconds when you are out of breath. Your doctor will suggest a treatment that can help you breathe properly and stop snoring.

Stress management

Chronic or persistent stress are the biggest risks for your brain, which can lead to shortening of your memory and hampering of your nerve cell growth. This leads to an increased risk of Alzheimer's disease and dementia. Manage the stress by putting yourself first; show some love and care for yourself by eating well, sleep enough, reduce the info you get via your social media, workout, and meditate.

One of the ways to reduce stress is to learn how to breathe properly. You now wonder how does one learn breathing? People tend to breathe shallow and fast. Spend at least ten minutes per day when you will breathe deeply. Provide your brain with enough oxygen and watch how all the stress reduces.

Find the time of your day to do relaxing things. Yes, work and life tend to cause us stress, but schedule time of the day when you will meditate, listen to relaxing music, practise yoga, or simply enjoy a good book.

Your inner peace is crucial for keeping stress away. No matter your religion, you can practice meditation, or if you feel more comfortable, you can pray and visit your local church or another object of worshiping.

Don't take things too seriously. Find time to have some fun and enjoy things such as dancing, reading, fishing, hiking, playing an instrument, playing cards with friends or family, do some gardening work, or do anything that makes you excited.

Laughter is the best medicine. Don't forget to laugh and include humor in your daily life. This includes even the ability to laugh at yourself.

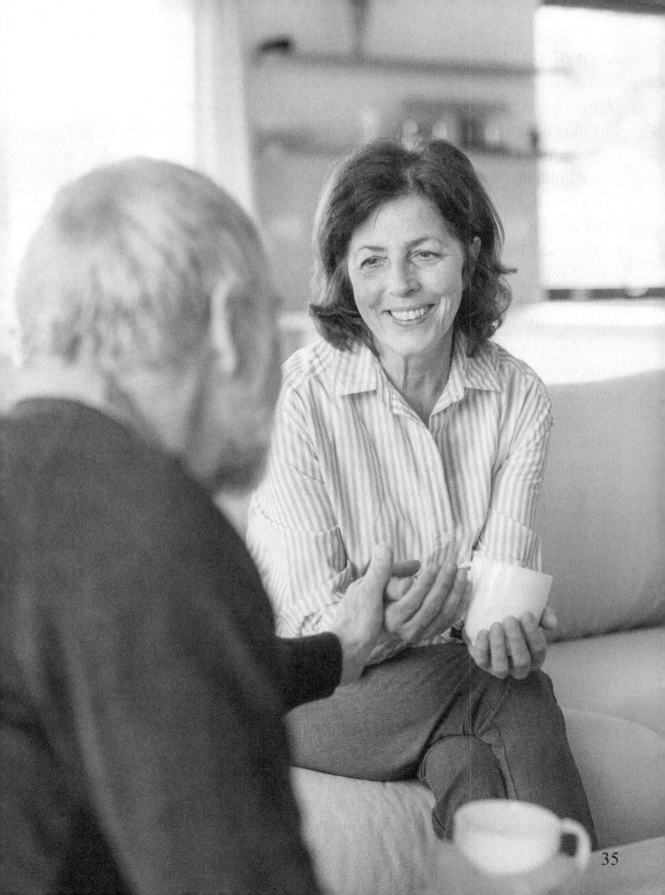

Keep Blood Pressure Under Control

Hypertension or high blood pressure is linked to a high risk of dementia. High blood pressure ruins tiny blood vessels in the parts of the brain that are responsible for cognition and memory.

Start checking your blood pressure regularly. Get a blood pressure device and check it at home. When you keep your blood pressure in track, you can be in control of taking responsibility to maintain it that way. If you can't get such a device, make sure to schedule a doctor appointment regularly so they can measure it for you.

Make changes in your diet and lifestyle. It does not matter if you were never good at working out or if you were always having issues with your weight. Now is always the right time to start. Keep your weight under control, start eating healthy foods, cut down cigarettes and coffee, limit your alcohol consummation one glass of red wine per day, and cut down the intake of sugar.

Takeout, processed, canned, and other junk food is not good for you, so it's time to cut the intake of such foods. High amounts of sugar and sodium are not friends of your health. Try to replace such foods with fresh vegetables and fruit. Make sure you are hydrated and drink at least eight glasses of water per day.

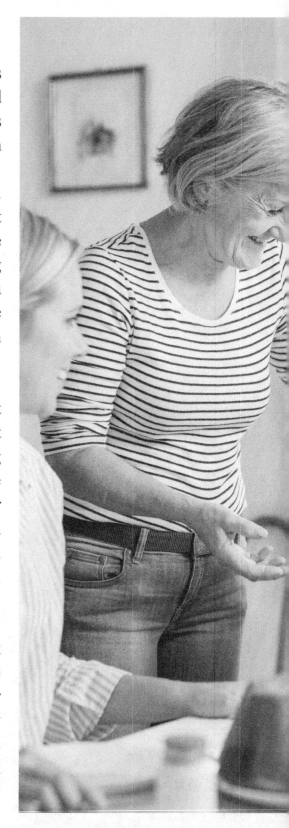

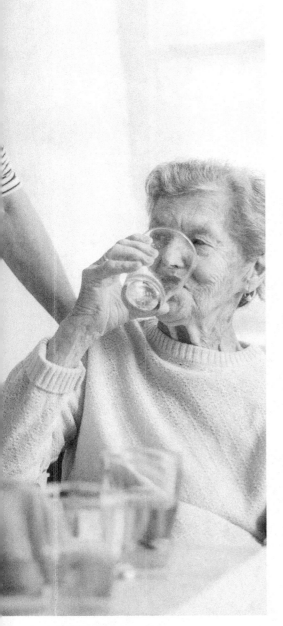

Don't forget to take the medication your doctor recommends. Prescribed medications are given to you with a purpose. When you keep your high blood pressure under control, your entire health will be in good shape.

Never ignore low blood pressure. Although it affects far fewer people, low blood pressure can reduce the blood flow in your brain. The main symptoms are blurred vision, dizziness, fatigue, unsteadiness when you stand up. Schedule a doctor's appointment if your blood pressure is constantly low.

Other Health Tips

It is not necessary to point out that smoking is severely damaging your health. Cutting this nasty habit is an excellent way to reduce the risk of Alzheimer's disease and dementia. Smokers over the age of sixty-five have almost 80% higher risk of this disease compared to people who don't' smoke. Keep your lungs free of smoke and breathe deeply for at least ten minutes a day.

Keep your cholesterol levels balanced. Studies suggest that there may be a link between high cholesterol and the risk for Alzheimer's and dementia. This is especially emphasized in people who have high cholesterol levels in their middle age.

37

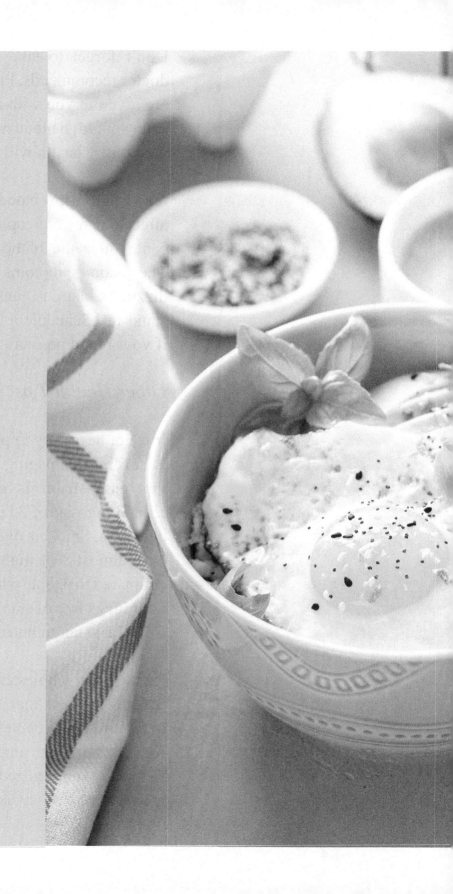

BREAKFAST RECIPES

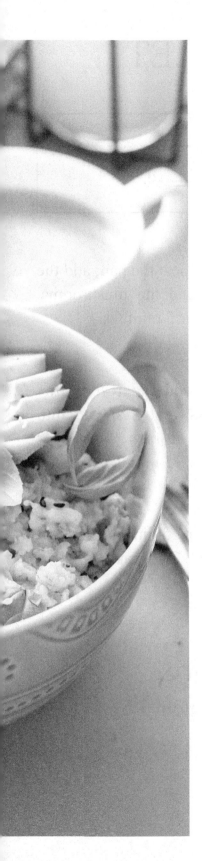
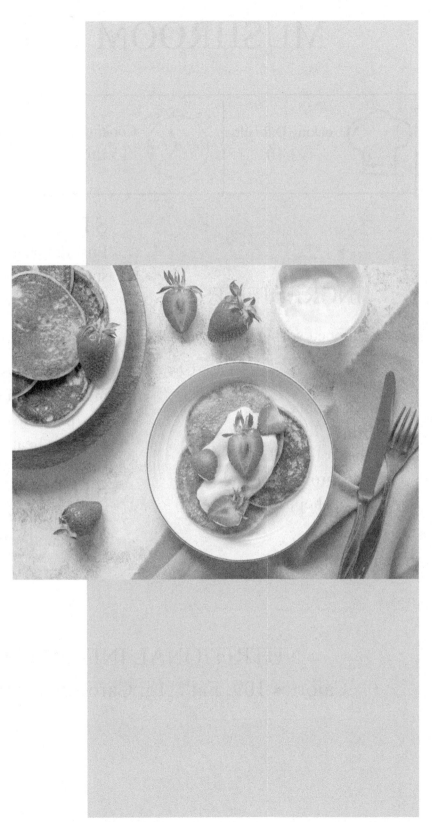

MUSHROOM OMELET

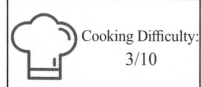 Cooking Difficulty: 3/10	Cooking Time: 15 minutes	Servings: 4

INGREDIENTS

- 2 chopped spring onions
- ½ lb. white mushrooms
- salt
- black pepper
- 4 whisked eggs
- 1 tbsp. olive oil
- ½ tsp. ground cumin
- 1 tbsp. chopped cilantro

STEP 1

Ensure that you heat the pan; add the spring onions and the mushrooms, toss and sauté for 5 minutes.

STEP 2

Add the eggs and the rest of the ingredients toss gently, spread into the pan, cover it then cook over medium heat for 15 minutes.

STEP 3

Slice the omelet, divide it between plates, and serve for breakfast.

NUTRITIONAL INFORMATION

Calories 109, Fat 8.1g, Carbs 2.9g, Protein 7.5g

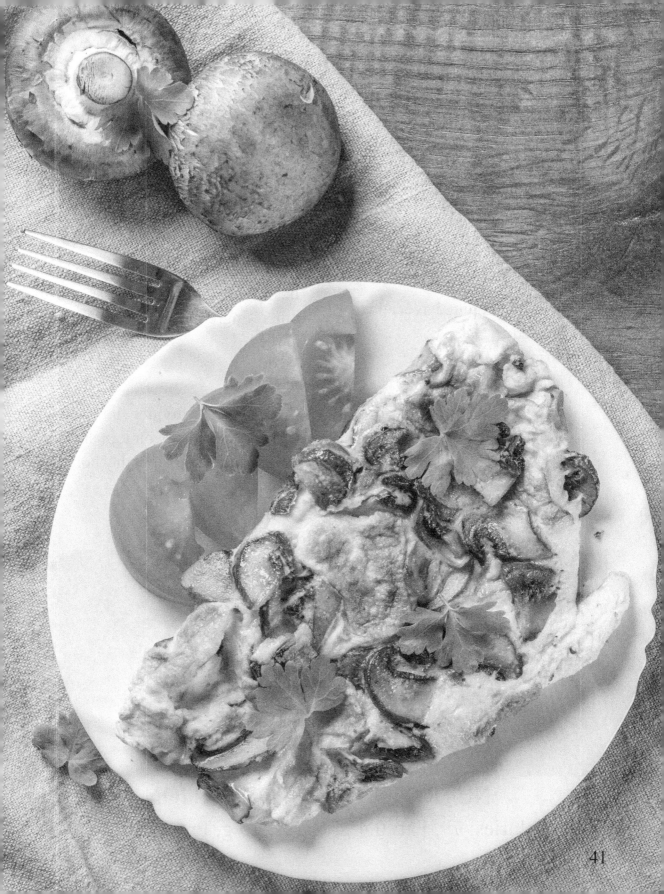

AVOCADO SPREAD

Cooking Difficulty: 1/10	Cooking Time: 1 minutes	Servings: 4

INGREDIENTS

- 2 peeled and pitted avocados, chopped
- 1 tbsp. olive oil
- 1 tbsp. minced shallots
- 1 tbsp. lime juice
- 1 tbsp. heavy coconut cream
- salt
- black pepper
- 1 tbsp. chopped chives

STEP 1

In a blender, combine the avocado flesh with the oil, shallots, and the other ingredients except for the chives.

STEP 2

Pulse well, divide into bowls, sprinkle the chives on top, and serve as a morning spread with whole grain bread.

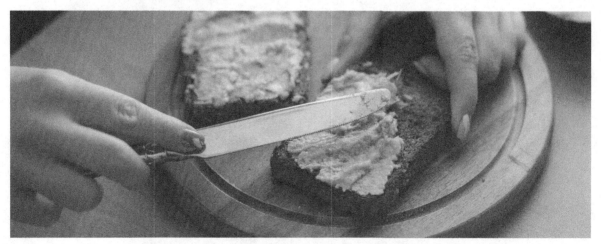

NUTRITIONAL INFORMATION
Calories: 79, Fat: 0.4 g, Carbs: 15 g, Protein: 1.3 g

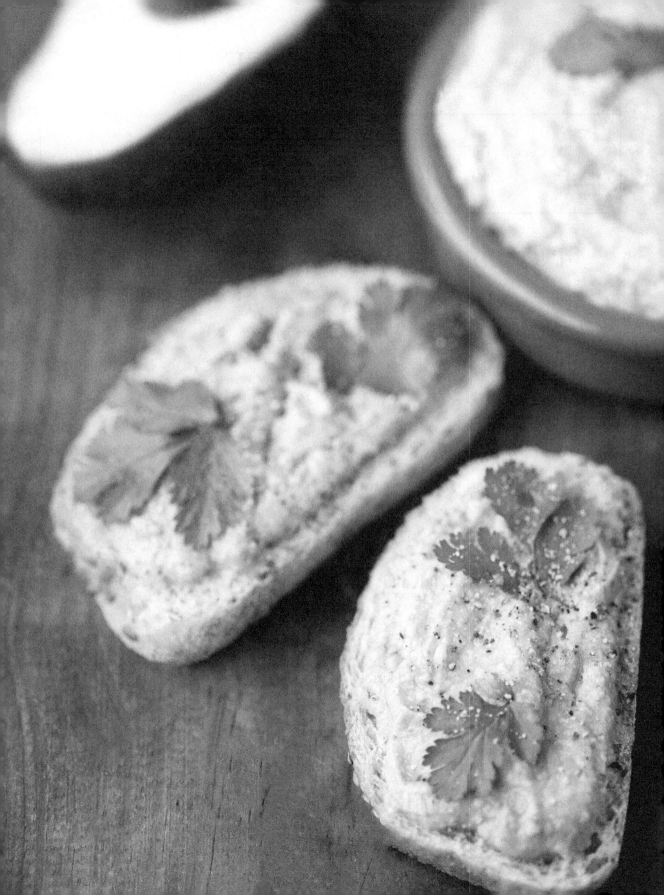

BEAN PATE

 Cooking Difficulty: 2/10

 Cooking Time: 10 minutes

 Servings: 4

INGREDIENTS

- 1 cup cooked beans
- 1 onion
- ½ glass of water
- 1 pinch of salt
- olive oil

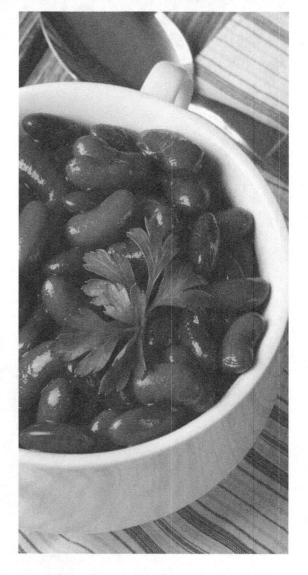

STEP 1
Finely chop the onion and fry until translucent.

STEP 2
Rinse the beans. Add oil and stir again.

STEP 3
Combine the onion, beans, and spices in a blender. If the consistency is not uniform, add water or oil. Serve with whole-grain bread.

NUTRITIONAL INFORMATION
Calories: 160; Fat: 3.6 g; Carbs: 17.1 g; Protein: 6.1 g

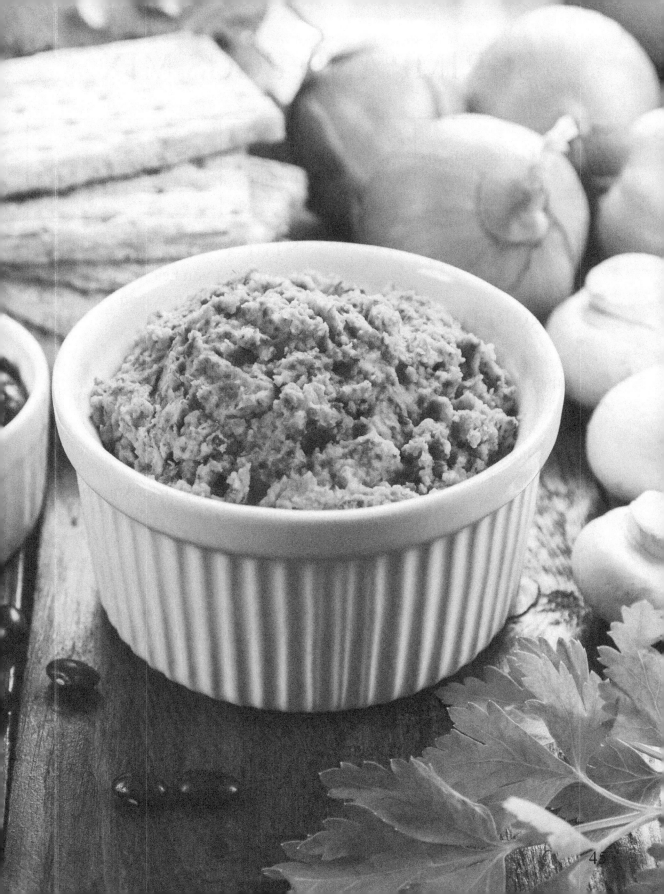

SHRIMP AND EGGS MIX

 Cooking Difficulty: 3/10

 Cooking Time: 13 minutes

 Servings: 4

INGREDIENTS

- 8 whisked eggs
- 1 tbsp. olive oil
- ½ lb. deveined shrimp, peeled and chopped
- ¼ c. chopped green onions
- 1 tsp. sweet paprika
- black pepper
- 1 tbsp. chopped cilantro

STEP 1
Ensure that you heat the pan; add the spring onions, toss and sauté for 2 minutes.

STEP 2
Add the shrimp, stir, then cook for 4 minutes more.

STEP 3
Add the eggs, paprika, salt, and pepper, toss, then cook for 5 minutes more.

STEP 4
Divide the mix between plates, sprinkle the cilantro on top, and serve for breakfast.

NUTRITIONAL INFORMATION
Calories 227, Fat 13.3g, Carbs 2.3g, Protein 24.2g

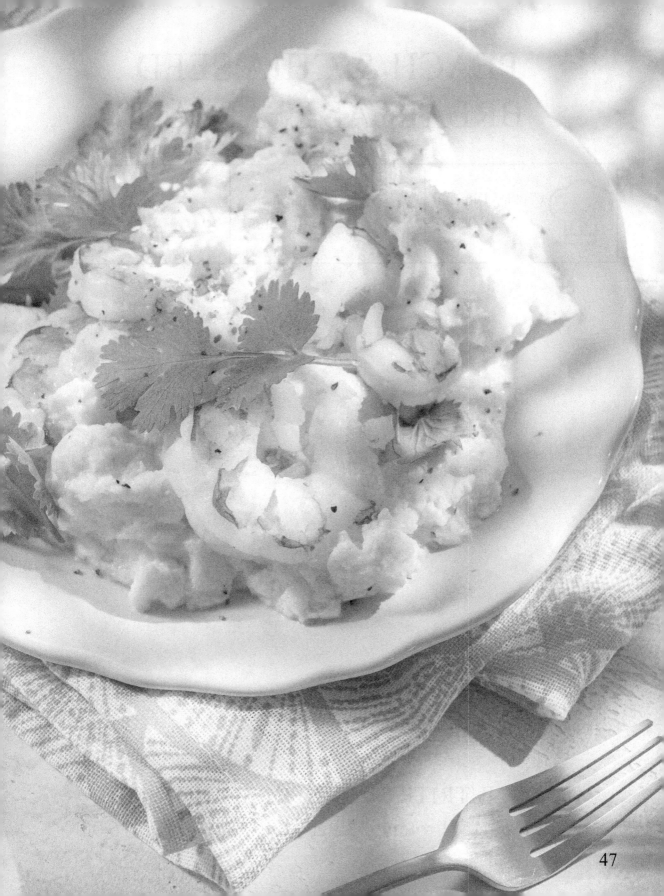

47

PEACH & CHIA SEED BREAKFAST PARFAIT

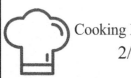 Cooking Difficulty:
2/10

 Cooking Time:
10 minutes

 Servings:
4

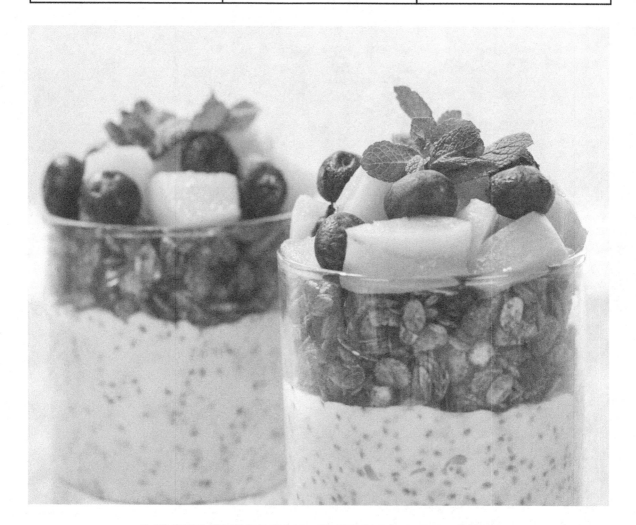

NUTRITIONAL INFORMATION
Calories: 415, Protein: 13.9g, Carbs: 54.4g, Fat: 16.9g

INGREDIENTS

- ½ oz. chia seeds
- 1 tbsp. pure maple syrup
- 1 c. coconut milk
- 1 tsp. ground cinnamon
- 3 diced peaches
- 2/3 c. granola

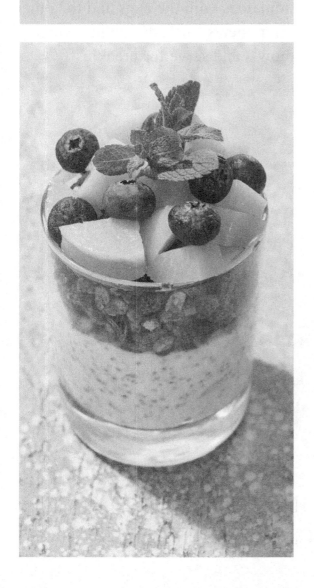

STEP 1

Find a small bowl and add the chia seeds, maple syrup, and coconut milk.

STEP 2

Stir well, then cover and pop into the fridge for at least one hour.

STEP 3

Find another bowl, add the peaches and sprinkle with the cinnamon. Pop to one side.

STEP 4

When it's time to serve, take two glasses, and pour the chia mixture between the two.

STEP 5

Sprinkle the granola over the top, keeping a tiny amount to one side to use to decorate later.

STEP 6

Top with the peaches and top with the reserved granola, optionally garnish with blueberries, and serve.

TOMATO AND EGGS SALAD

Cooking Difficulty: 1/10	Cooking Time: 3 minutes	Servings: 4

INGREDIENTS

- 4 hard-boiled eggs, peeled and chopped
- 2 c. halved cherry tomatoes
- 1 c. pitted kalamata olives halved
- 1 c. arugula or spinach
- 2 chopped spring onions
- black pepper
- 1 tbsp. avocado oil

STEP 1

In a salad bowl, combine the tomatoes with the eggs and the other ingredients, toss, divide into smaller bowls and serve for breakfast.

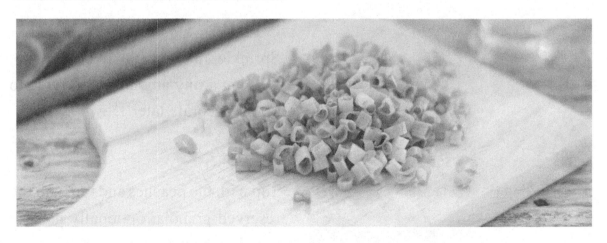

NUTRITIONAL INFORMATION
Calories 126, Fat 8.6g, Carbs 6.9g, Protein 6.9g

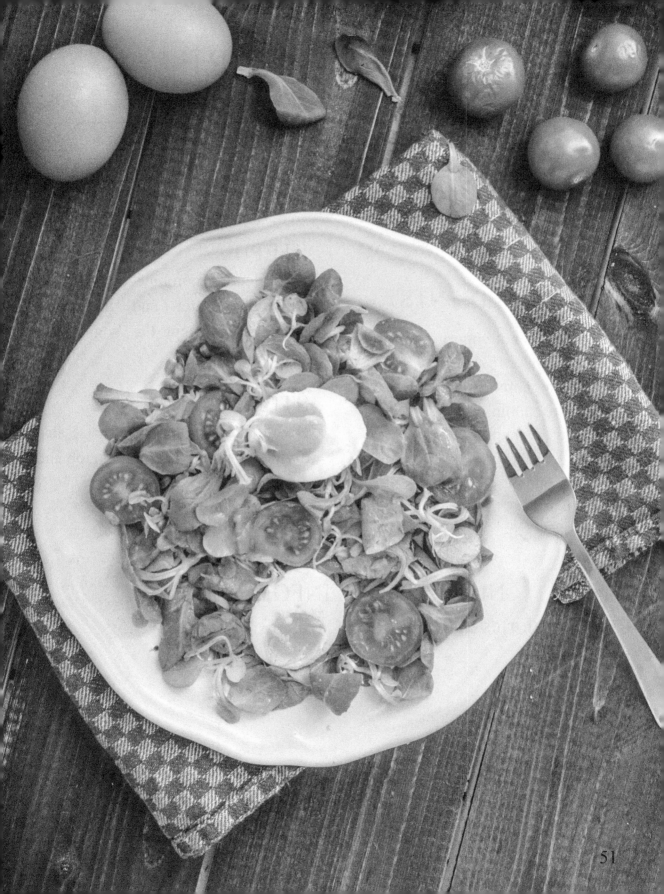

PEACHES AND CREAM

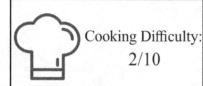 Cooking Difficulty: 2/10

 Cooking Time: 4 minutes

 Servings: 4

INGREDIENTS

- 2 c. coconut yogurt
- ½ c. water
- 1 pear, cored and chopped
- 2 tsps. pumpkin pie spice
- 2 tbsps. maple syrup
- ¼ c. cashews
- 2 c. pumpkin puree

STEP 1

In a blender, combine the cashews with the water and the other ingredients except the yogurt and pulse well.

STEP 2

Divide the yogurt into bowls, also divide the pumpkin cream on top and serve.

NUTRITIONAL INFORMATION

Calories 200, Fat 6.4g, Carbs 32.9g, Protein 5.5g

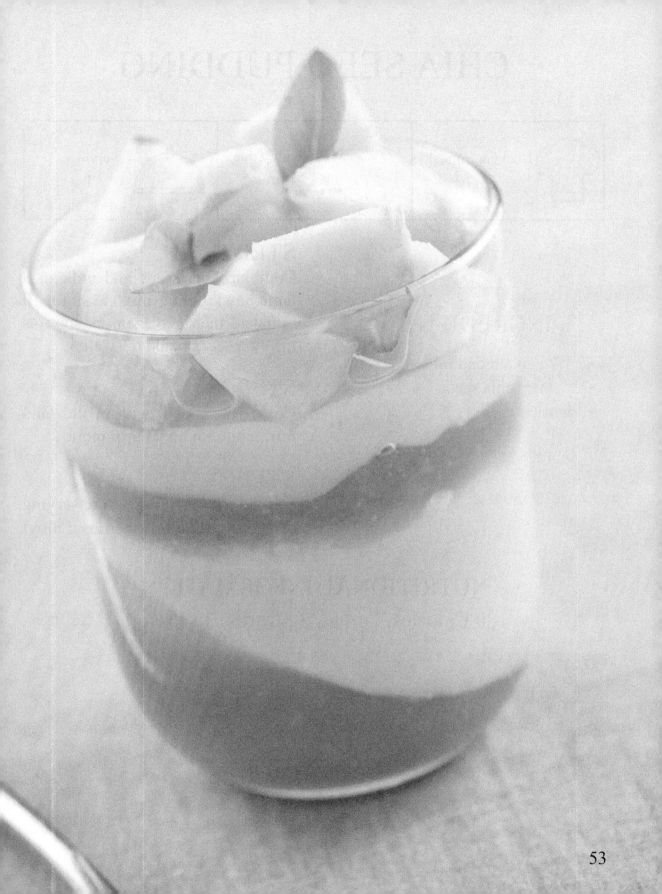

CHIA SEED PUDDING

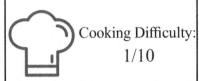 Cooking Difficulty: 1/10	Cooking Time: 12 minutes	Servings: 1

INGREDIENTS

- 1/2 cup almond milk
- 2 tbsp. chia seeds
- berries

STEP 1

Combine chia seeds and milk in a large bowl. Let the mixture sit for 10 minutes, then stir again as soon as the chia seeds begin to swell.

STEP 2

Cover the bowl with a lid and refrigerate for an hour or more.

STEP 3

Stir the chia pudding before serving and add your favorite berries. Enjoy!

NUTRITIONAL INFORMATION

180 Calories, 7g Fat, 3g Carbs, 3g Protein

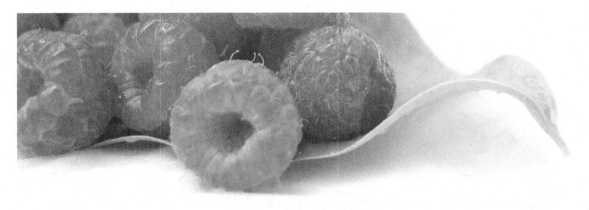

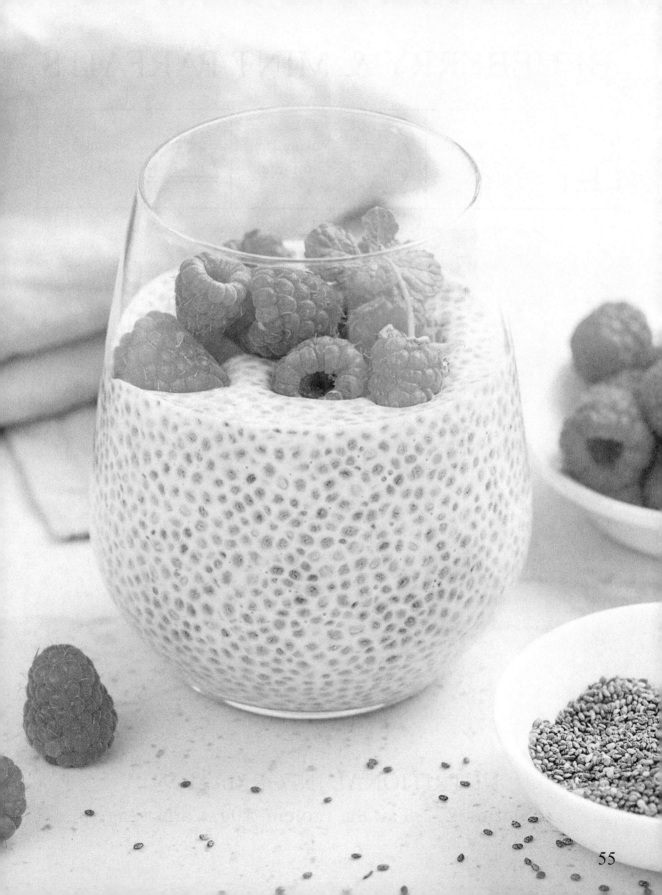

BLUEBERRY & MINT PARFAITS

Cooking Difficulty: 2/10	Cooking Time: 5 minutes	Servings: 4

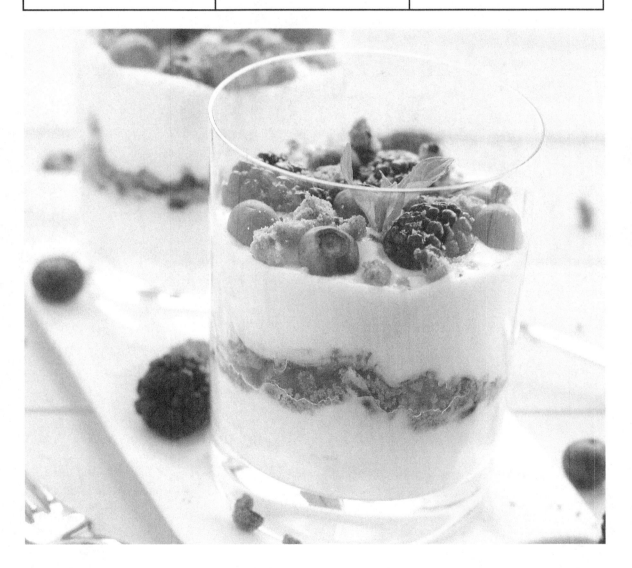

NUTRITIONAL INFORMATION
Calories: 272, Fat: 8g, Protein: 10g, Carbs: 25g

INGREDIENTS

- 1½ c. wholegrain rolled oats
- 1 c. almond milk
- 2 c. Greek yogurt, unsweetened
- 1 c. fresh blueberries
- blackberries (optional)
- 4 freshly chopped mint leaves

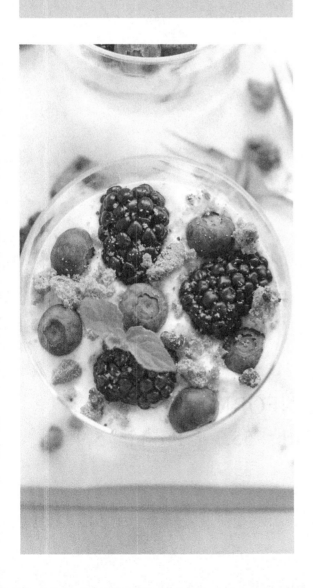

STEP 1
Place the oats and almond milk into a bowl and stir together to combine (this helps the oats to soften).

STEP 2
Spoon the oat and almond milk mixture evenly into your 4 containers.

STEP 3
Place a drop of yogurt into each container on top of the oats (use half of the yogurt as you'll be adding another layer of it).

STEP 4
Divide half of the blueberries between the 4 containers and sprinkle on top of the yogurt.

STEP 5
Add another layer of yogurt and then another layer of blueberries (you can use them all up at this stage).

STEP 6
Sprinkle the fresh mint over the top of each parfait.

STEP 7
Cover and place into the fridge to store until needed!

KIWI SPINACH SMOOTHIE

Cooking Difficulty: 1/10	Cooking Time: 1 minutes	Servings: 1

INGREDIENTS

- 1 c. baby spinach
- 2 peeled kiwi, halved
- ½ c. apple juice
- 2 tbsps. flaxseed, ground
- ½ peeled banana
- 12 ice cubes

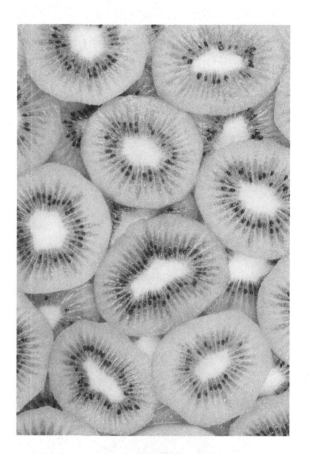

STEP 1

Using a blender, set in all your ingredients. Blend well until very smooth. Enjoy!

NUTRITIONAL INFORMATION
Calories: 284, Fat: 5.6 g, Carbs: 55.3 g, Protein: 5.9 g

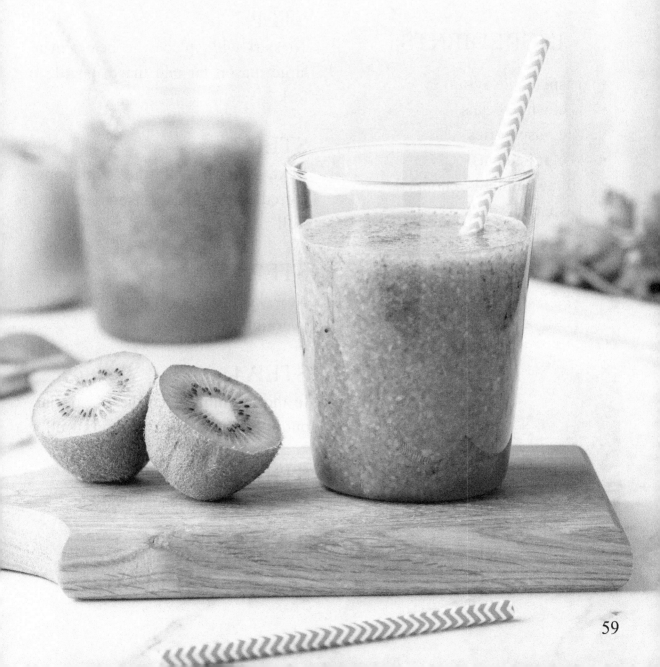

RASPBERRY OVERNIGHT OATS

 Cooking Difficulty: 2/10

 Cooking Time: 5 minutes

 Servings: 2

INGREDIENTS

- 1 tsp. maple syrup
- ¼ c. white beans
- ¼ c. raspberries
- ½ c. rolled oats
- 10 raw almonds, chopped
- 1 tsp. chia seeds
- 2/3 c. soy milk

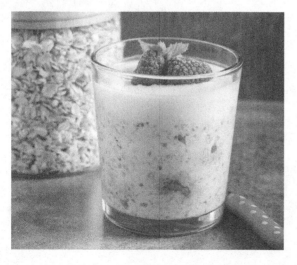

STEP 1
To start with, place the beans in a large mason jar and mash it with a fork.

STEP 2
Next, stir in all the remaining ingredients to the Mason jar. Mix well.

STEP 3
Now, keep the jar in the refrigerator overnight.

STEP 4
In the morning, keep the Mason jar out of the refrigerator and mix well.

STEP 5
Serve immediately and enjoy it.

NUTRITIONAL INFORMATION
Calories: 371, Proteins: 16.8g, Carbs: 54.5g, Fat: 11.4g

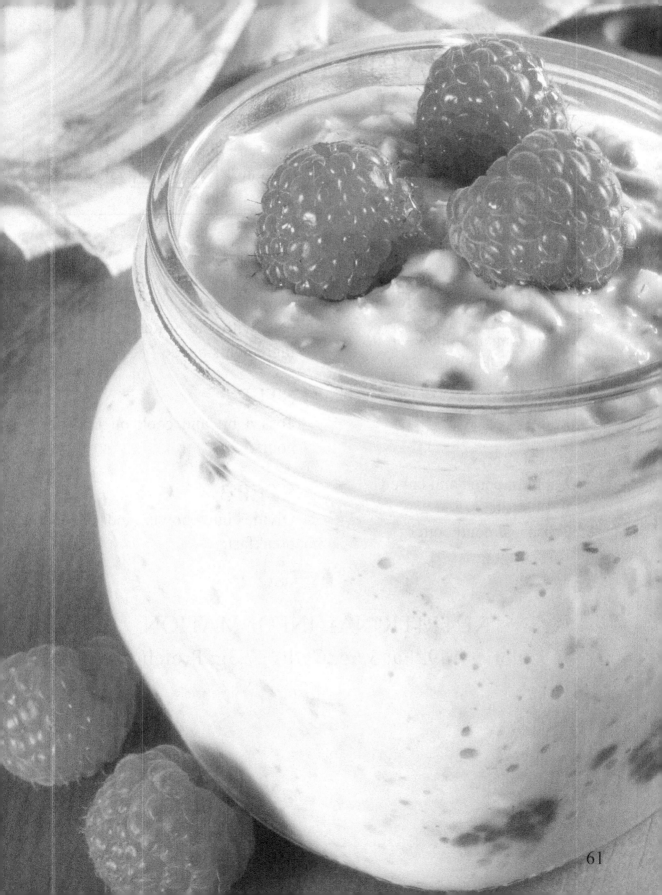

APPLE OATS

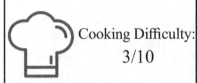 Cooking Difficulty: 3/10	Cooking Time: 420 minutes	Servings: 4

INGREDIENTS

- ½ tsp. cinnamon powder
- 1 ½ c. almond milk
- 1 c. oats, gluten-free
- 1 tbsp. flax seed, ground
- 2 tbsps. swerve
- cooking spray
- 2 apples, cored and cubed
- 1 ½ c. water
- 2 tbsps. almond butter

STEP 1
Grease a slow cooker with the cooking spray and combine the oats with the water and the other ingredients inside.

STEP 2
Toss a bit and cook on Low for 7 hours.

STEP 3
Divide into bowls and serve for breakfast.

NUTRITIONAL INFORMATION
Calories 149, Fat 3.6g, Carbs 27.3g, Protein 4.9g

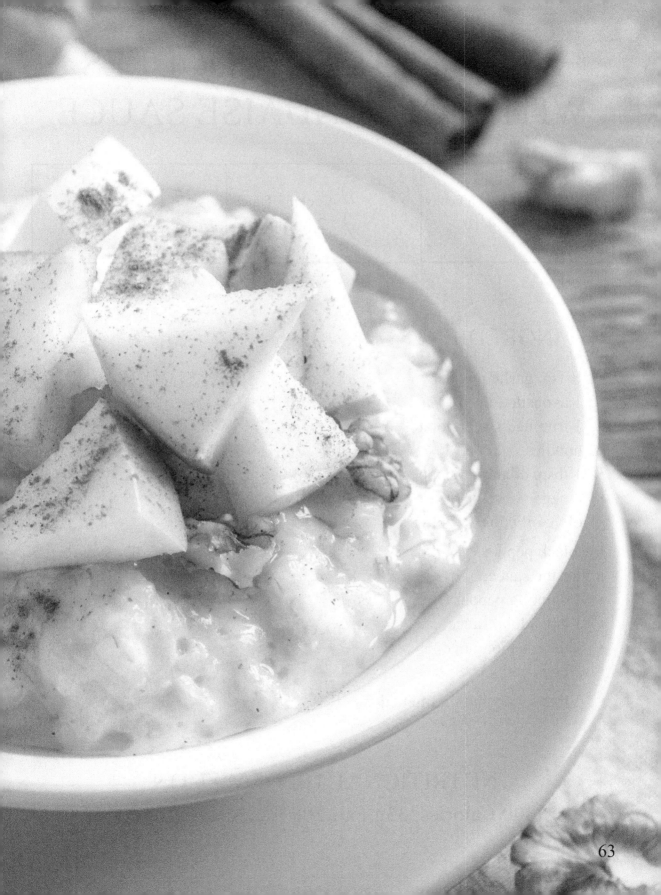

SWEET POTATO NOODLES WITH HOLLANDAISE SAUCE

 Cooking Difficulty: 4/10

 Cooking Time: 20 minutes

 Servings: 3

INGREDIENTS

- ¼ tsp. garlic powder
- 1 avocado, diced
- 1 trimmed sweet potato, noodles
- 1 tbsp. cilantro, chopped
- 3 eggs
- olive oil cooking spray
- black pepper
for the sauce:
- 1 chipotle pepper
- 1 tsp. adobo sauce
- 1 tbsp. lemon juice
- 2 eggs yolks
- 3 tbsps. coconut oil, melted

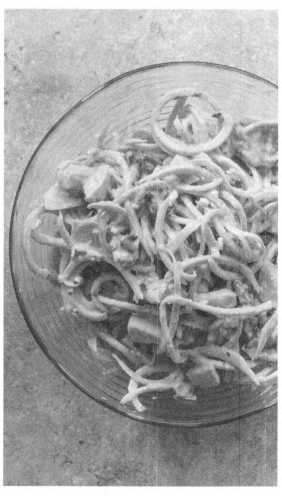

NUTRITIONAL INFORMATION
400 Calories, 33g Fat, 20g Carbs, 11g Protein

STEP 1

Pre-heat your oven to 425 Degrees Fahrenheit. Lightly coat with cooking spray a baking sheet, place the sweet potato noodle and season it with pepper and garlic powder. Sprinkle avocado cubes on top and roast until the sweet potato noodles are cooked or for around 10 to 13 minutes.

STEP 2

Meanwhile, place the lemon juice, sauce, egg yolks, and chipotle pepper in a blender and pulse for around 10 seconds. Then, put the blender on medium and gradually add the coconut oil to thicken. Set aside. Once done with the hollandaise sauce, pour water in a medium saucepan fill it halfway and simmer.

STEP 3

Break the eggs into a small bowl or ramekin. Then, make a gentle whirlpool in the simmering water so the egg white will wrap around the yolk. Gradually tip the egg into the water. Cook for 3 mins. Remove eggs from water by use of a slotted spoon and transfer it on a paper towel-lined plate.

STEP 4

As soon as the avocado and sweet potato noodles are done, make a nest on 3 plates. Place poached eggs on top and drizzle with hollandaise sauce. Serve and garnish it with cilantro.

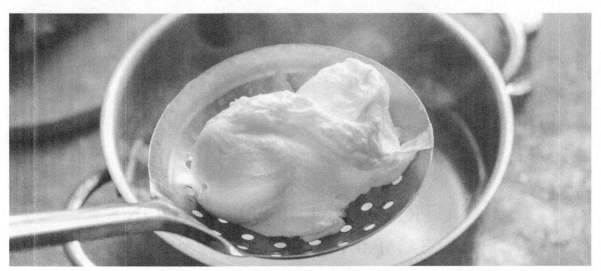

SPINACH OMELET

Cooking Difficulty: 2/10	Cooking Time: 20 minutes	Servings: 4

INGREDIENTS

- 8 whisked eggs
- 1 c. baby spinach
- salt
- black pepper
- 1 tbsp. olive oil
- 2 chopped spring onions
- 1 tsp. sweet paprika
- 1 tsp. ground cumin
- 1 tbsp. chopped chives

STEP 1
Ensure that you heat the pan; add the spring onions, paprika, and cumin, stir and sauté for 5 minutes.

STEP 2
Add the eggs, the spinach, salt, and pepper toss spread into the pan, cover it then cook for 15 minutes.

STEP 3
Sprinkle the chives on top, divide everything between plates and serve.

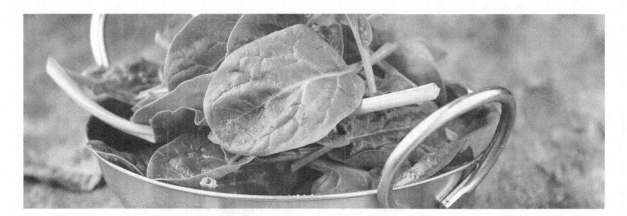

NUTRITIONAL INFORMATION
Calories 345, Fat 12g, Carbs 8g, Protein 13.3g

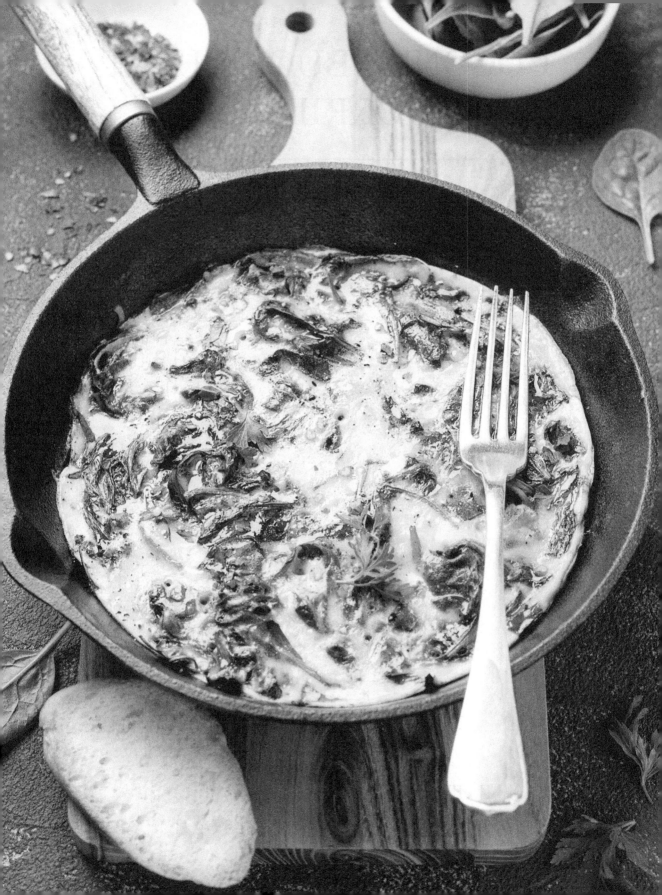

COCONUT BUCKWHEAT PORRIDGE

Cooking Difficulty: 2/10	Cooking Time: 12 minutes	Servings: 6

INGREDIENTS

- 1 c. water
- 2 tsps. vanilla extract
- 1 c. buckwheat grouts
- dash of salt
- ¼ c. chia seeds
- ¼ tsp. cinnamon
- 3 c. unsweetened coconut milk

STEP 1
For making this high-protein porridge, you need to mix all the ingredients in a large mixing bowl until combined well.

STEP 2
Then, cover the bowl with plastic cling and place it in the refrigerator overnight.

STEP 3
Next morning, transfer the contents to a deep saucepan over medium heat.

STEP 4
Cook for 10 minutes or until thickened. Tip: Make sure to stir it continuously. Serve it hot or warm.

NUTRITIONAL INFORMATION
Calories: 387, Proteins: 7g, Carbs: 25.3g, Fat: 31.4g

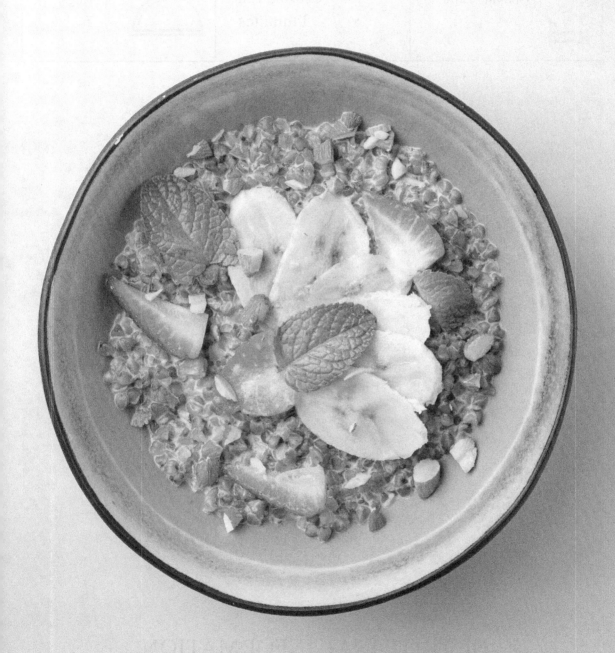

CHICKPEA COOKIE DOUGH

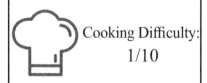 Cooking Difficulty: 1/10

 Cooking Time: 3 minutes

 Servings: 6

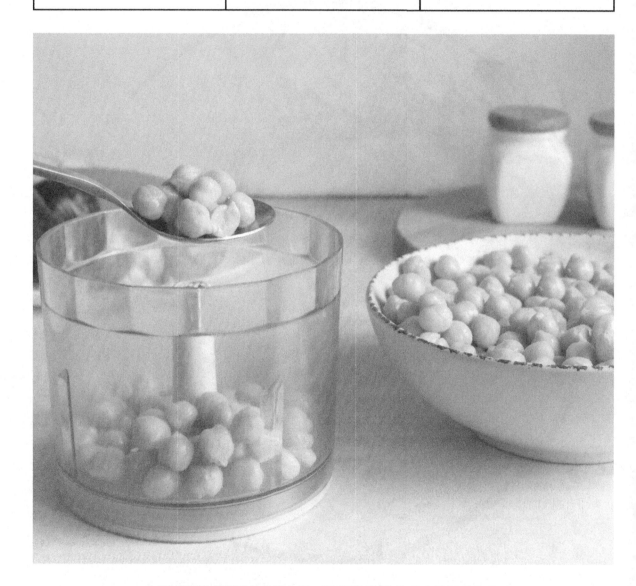

NUTRITIONAL INFORMATION
Calories: 415, Protein: 13.9g, Carbs: 54.4g, Fat: 16.9g

INGREDIENTS

- ½ tsp. sea salt
- 2 c. cooked chickpeas, drained
- ¼ c. maple syrup
- 1/3 c. melted coconut oil
- 3 tbsps. coconut flour
- 2 tsps. vanilla extract

STEP 1

To make this delightful cookie dough, first, blend the chickpeas in a high-speed blender for a minute or until smooth.

STEP 2

Spoon in the oil, sea salt, maple syrup, and vanilla extract. Blend for a further minute or until combined.

STEP 3

Next, stir in the coconut flour and blend again. Scrape the sides.

STEP 4

Now, transfer the mixture to a medium-sized bowl and place in the refrigerator for 2 hours. Serve on its own or with crackers.

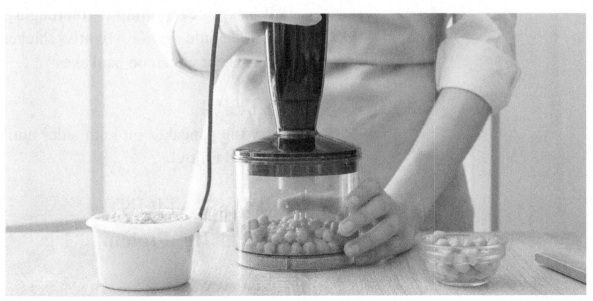

SPINACH PANCAKES

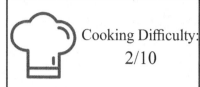 Cooking Difficulty: 2/10	Cooking Time: 15 minutes	Servings: 2

INGREDIENTS

- 0.5 glass coconut milk
- 1 cup flour
- 2 egg
- 3 tbsp. coconut oil
- ½ teaspoon baking soda
- ½ teaspoon salt
- spinach

STEP 1
Dip the spinach leaves in boiling water for 3-5 seconds, then remove and transfer to ice water.

STEP 2
Put the spinach leaves treated with boiling water in a blender, add eggs and milk, beat on high speed until smooth.

STEP 3
Add flour, salt, soda, oil to a blender. Whisk everything thoroughly. You should get a slightly thicker consistency than on pancakes.

STEP 4
Fry the pancakes on both sides until tender. Enjoy!

NUTRITIONAL INFORMATION
Calories: 190; Fat: 1.3 g; Carbs: 11.1 g; Protein: 2.1 g

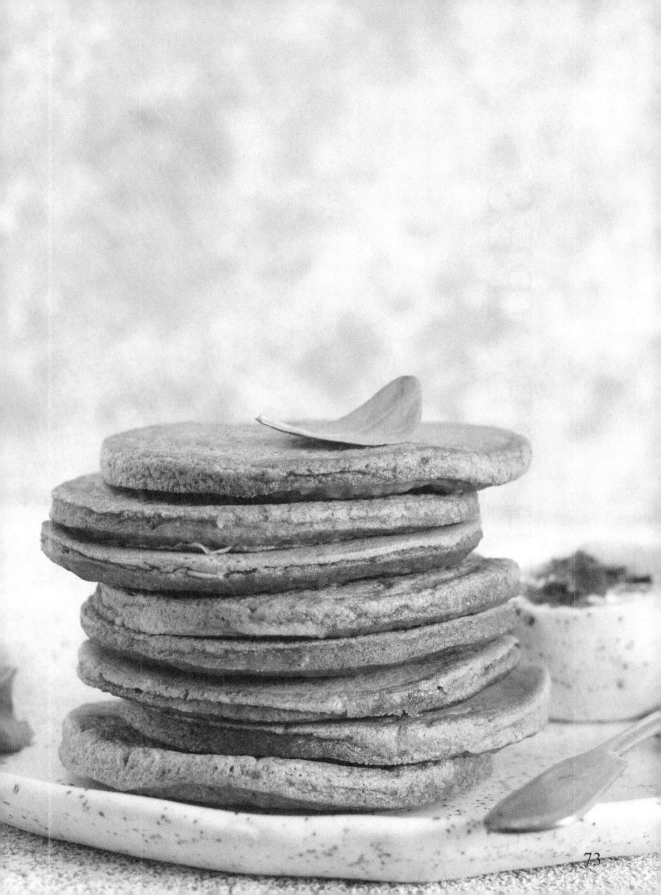

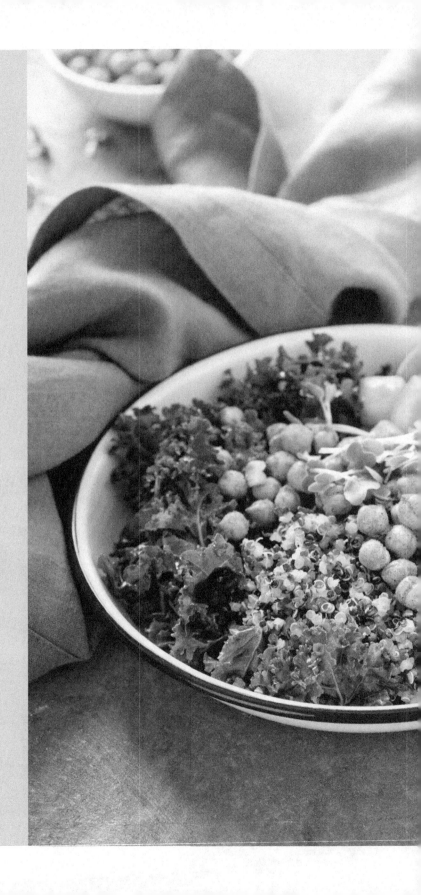

LUNCH RECIPES

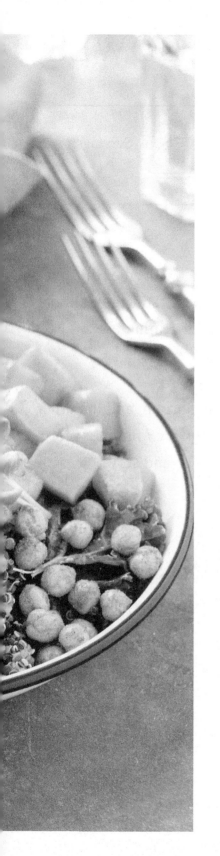

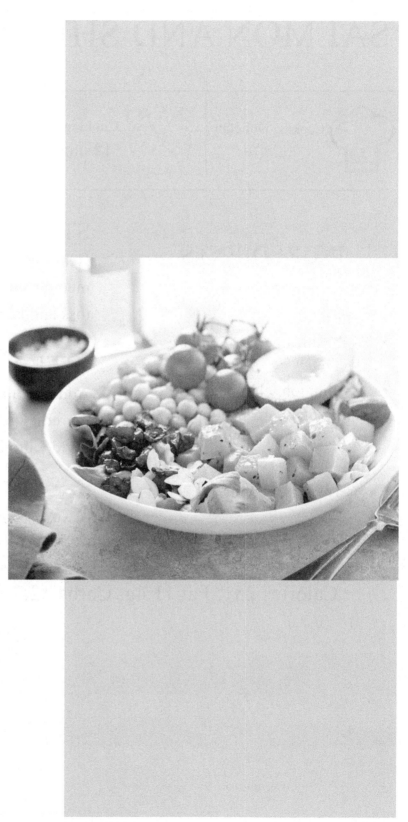

SALMON AND SHRIMP BOWLS

Cooking Difficulty: 2/10	Cooking Time: 12 minutes	Servings: 4

INGREDIENTS

- ½ c. mild salsa
- 1 tbsp. olive oil
- ½ lb. shrimp, peeled and deveined
- 1 red onion, chopped
- 2 tbsps. cilantro, chopped
- ½ lb. smoked salmon, skinless, deboned and cubed
- ¼ c. tomatoes, cubed

STEP 1

Heat up a pan with the oil over medium-high heat, add the salmon, toss and cook for 5 minutes.

STEP 2

Add the onion, shrimp, and the other ingredients, cook for 7 minutes more, divide into bowls, and serve.

NUTRITIONAL INFORMATION
Calories 251, Fat 11.4g, Carbs 12.3g, Protein 7.1g

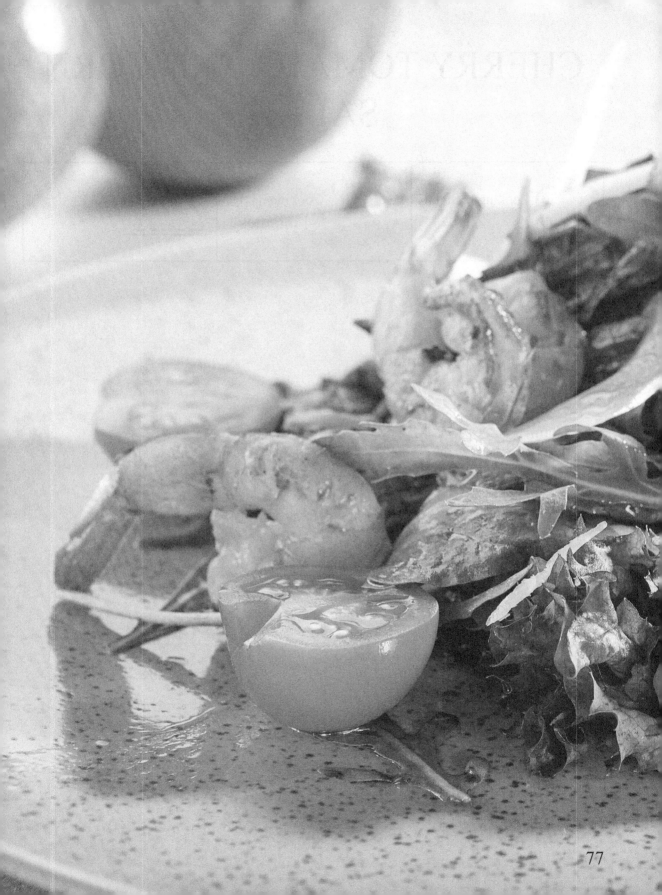

CHERRY TOMATO AND CORN SALAD

Cooking Difficulty: 2/10	Cooking Time: 4 minutes	Servings: 2

INGREDIENTS

- 1 branch of cherry tomatoes
- 1 can of canned corn
- 3 avocados
- cilantro
- lemon juice
- salt pepper

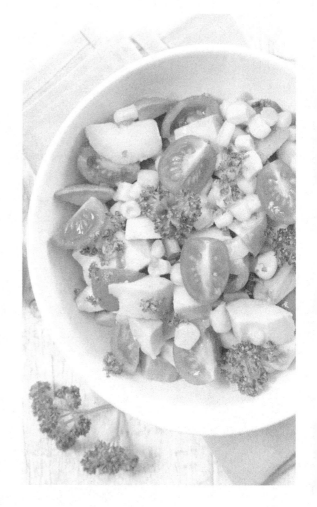

STEP 1
Chop tomatoes, cilantro, and avocado.

STEP 2
Mix in a salad bowl with corn, season with lemon juice, and add spices.

STEP 3
Divide the salad into plates.

NUTRITIONAL INFORMATION
Calories 99, Fat 3.8g, Carbs 11.5g, Protein 4.9g

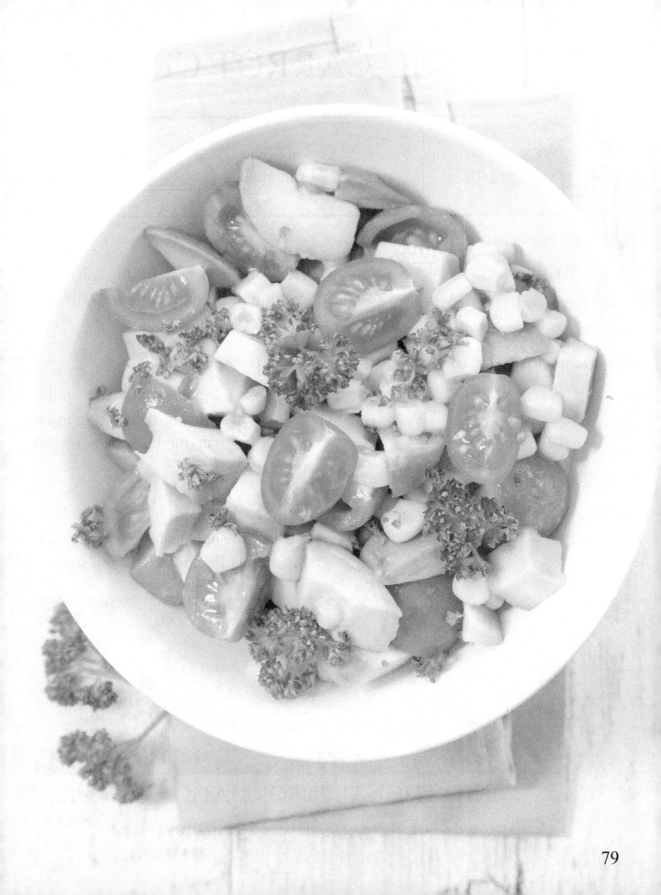

TURMERIC CARROT CREAM

Cooking Difficulty: 2/10	Cooking Time: 24 minutes	Servings: 4

INGREDIENTS

- 5 c. chicken stock, low-sodium
- 1 lb. carrots, peeled and chopped
- 2 tbsps. olive oil
- 4 celery stalks, chopped
- ¼ tsp. black pepper
- 1 tbsp. cilantro, chopped
- 1 yellow onion, chopped
- 1 tsp. turmeric powder

STEP 1
Heat up a pot with the oil over medium heat, add the onion, stir and sauté for 2 minutes.

STEP 2
Add the carrots and the other ingredients, bring to a simmer, and cook over medium heat for 20 minutes.

STEP 3
Blend the soup using an immersion blender, ladle into bowls and serve.

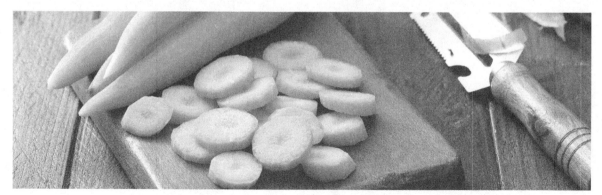

NUTRITIONAL INFORMATION
Calories 221, Fat 9.6g, Carbs 16g, Protein 4.8g

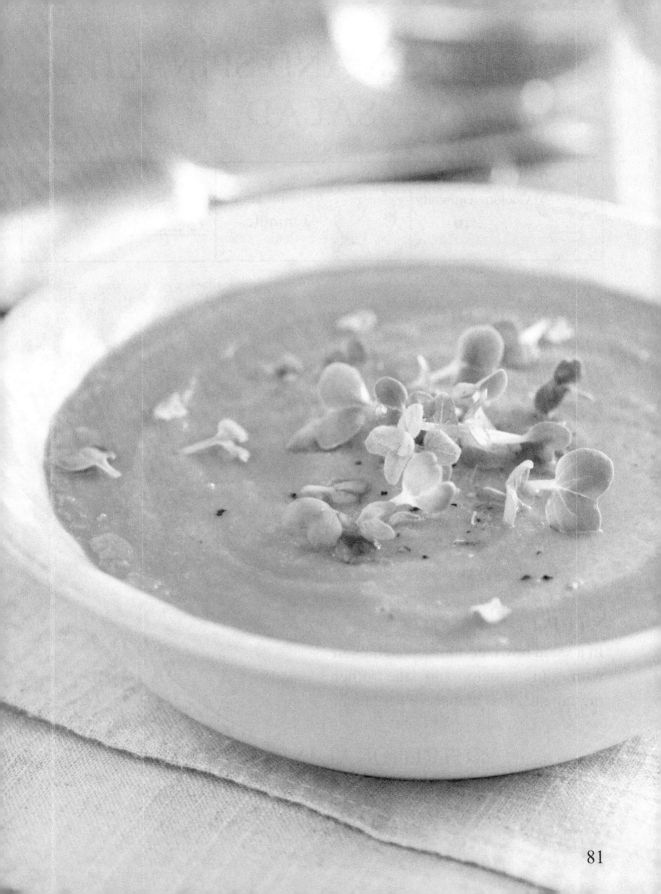

CHICKEN AND SPINACH SALAD

Cooking Difficulty: 2/10	Cooking Time: 3 minutes	Servings: 4

INGREDIENTS

- ¼ tsp. black pepper
- 1 red onion, chopped
- 2 rotisserie chicken, de-boned, skinless and shredded
- ¼ c. walnuts, chopped
- 1 lb. cherry tomatoes, halved
- green pea
- 2 tbsps. lemon juice
- 1 tbsp. olive oil
- 4 c. baby spinach

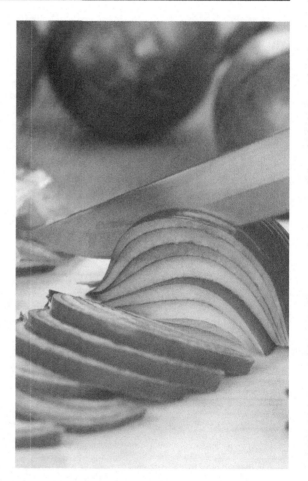

STEP 1

In a salad bowl, combine the chicken with the tomato and the other ingredients, toss and serve for lunch.

NUTRITIONAL INFORMATION
Calories 380, Fat 40g, Carbs 1g, Protein 17g

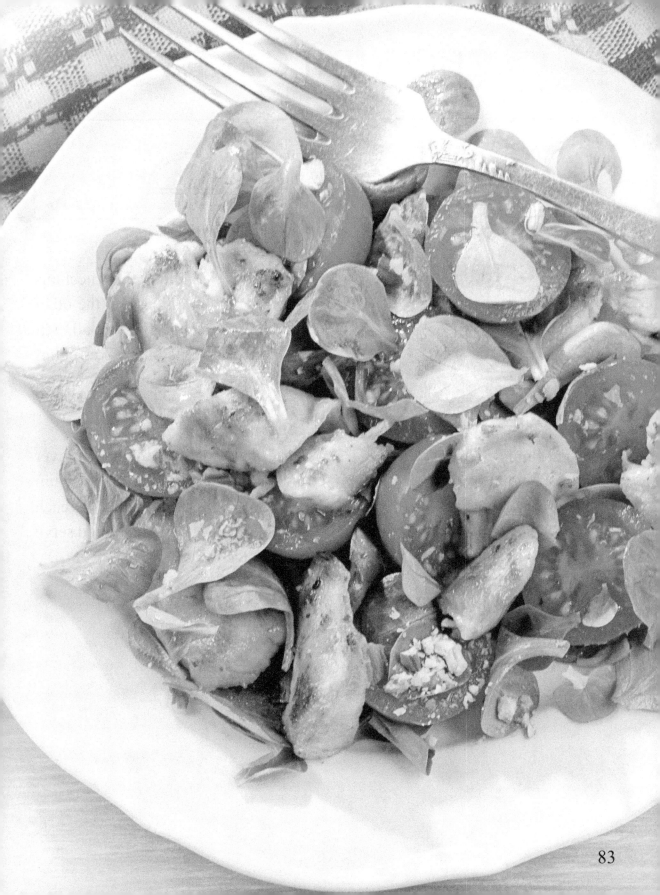

ZUCCHINI CAKES

Cooking Difficulty: 2/10	Cooking Time: 22 minutes	Servings: 4

INGREDIENTS

- 2 tbsps. olive oil
- 2 tbsps. almond flour
- 1/3 c. carrot, shredded
- 1 tsp. lemon zest, grated
- 1 garlic clove, minced
- 1 egg, whisked
- 2 zucchinis, grated
- 1 tbsp. cilantro, chopped
- 1 yellow onion, chopped
- ¼ tsp. black pepper
- salt

STEP 1

In a bowl, combine the zucchinis with the garlic, onion, and the other ingredients except for the oil, stir well and shape medium cakes out of this mix.

STEP 2

Heat up a pan with the oil over medium-high heat, add the zucchini cakes, cook for 5 minutes on each side, divide between plates and serve with a side salad.

NUTRITIONAL INFORMATION
Calories 271, Fat 8.7g, Carbs 14.3g, Protein 4.6g

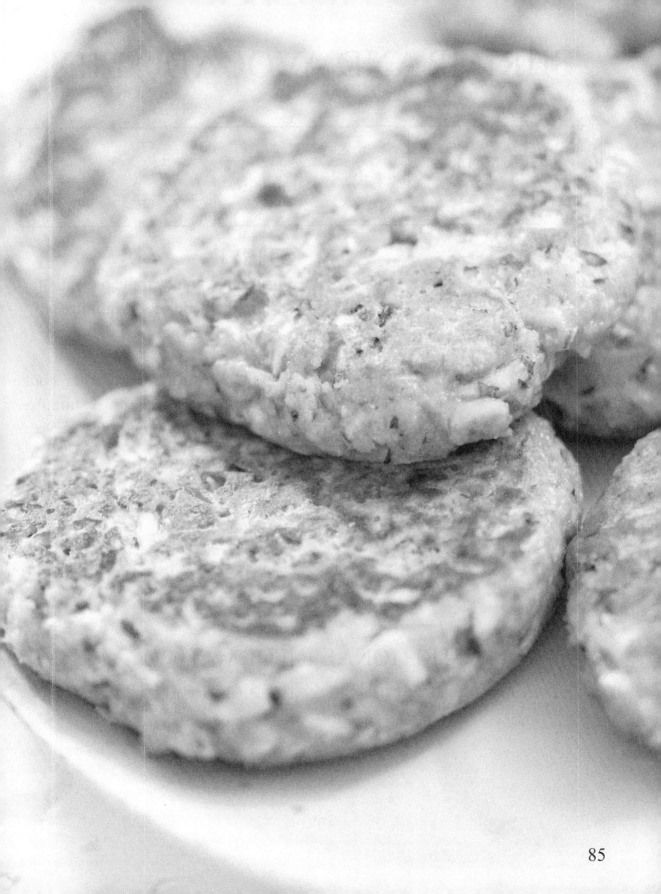

SHRIMP AND AVOCADO MIX

 Cooking Difficulty:
2/10

 Cooking Time:
8 minutes

 Servings:
4

INGREDIENTS

- 1 lb. peeled shrimp, deveined
- 1 tbsp. avocado oil
- ½ c. chopped arugula
- salt
- black pepper
- 1 pitted avocado, peeled
- 2 tbsps. lime juice
- 2 tbsps. chopped parsley

STEP 1
Ensure that you heat the pan, add the shrimp then cook for 4 minutes.

STEP 2
Add the rest of the ingredients, cook over medium heat for 3 minutes more, divide into bowls, and serve.

NUTRITIONAL INFORMATION
Calories 240, Fat 12g, Carbs 5.6g, Protein 25g

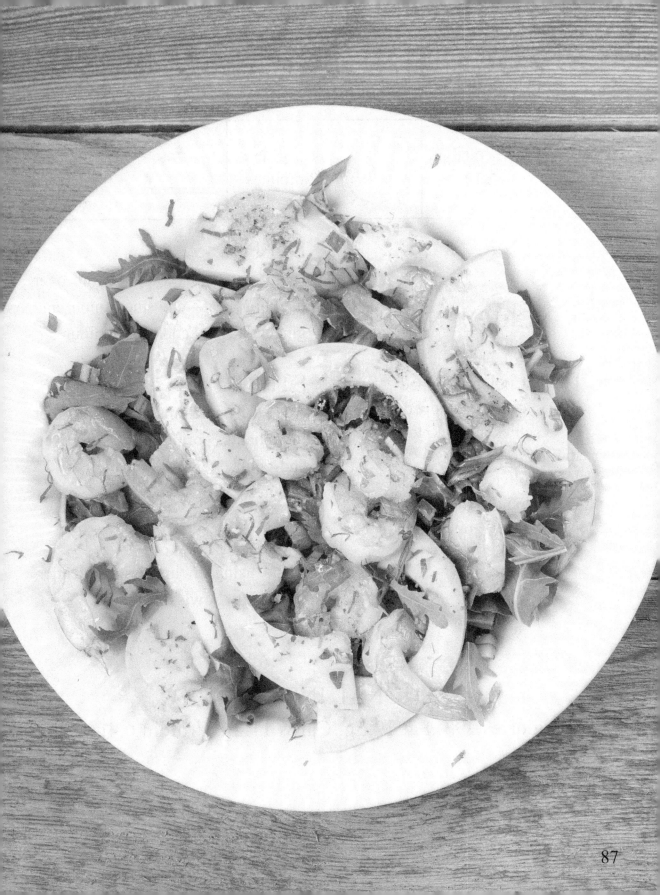

ZUCCHINI CREAM SOUP

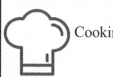 Cooking Difficulty: 2/10	Cooking Time: 22 minutes	Servings: 4

INGREDIENTS

- 1 tbsp. dill, chopped
- 1 yellow onion, chopped
- 1 lb. zucchinis, chopped
- 32 oz. chicken stock, low-sodium
- 1 tbsp. olive oil
- 1 c. coconut cream
- 1 tsp. ginger, grated

STEP 1

Heat up a pot with the oil over medium heat, add the onion and ginger, stir and cook for 5 minutes.

STEP 2

Add the zucchinis and the other ingredients, bring to a simmer, and cook over medium heat for 15 minutes.

STEP 3

Blend using an immersion blender, divide into bowls and serve.

NUTRITIONAL INFORMATION

Calories 293, Fat 12.3g, Carbs 11.2g, Protein 6.4g

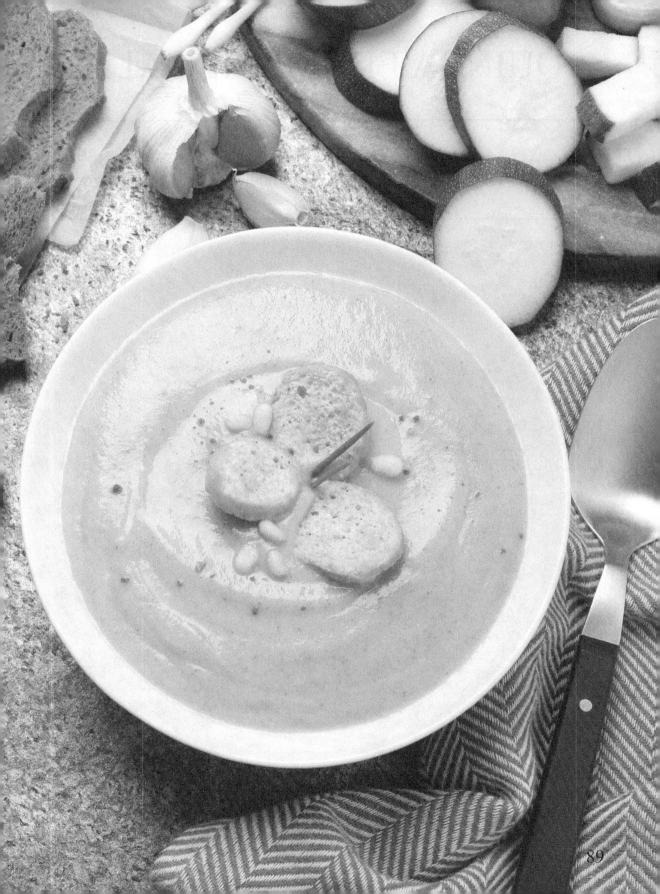

QUINOA EDAMAME SALAD

 Cooking Difficulty:
3/10

 Cooking Time:
25 minutes

 Servings:
4

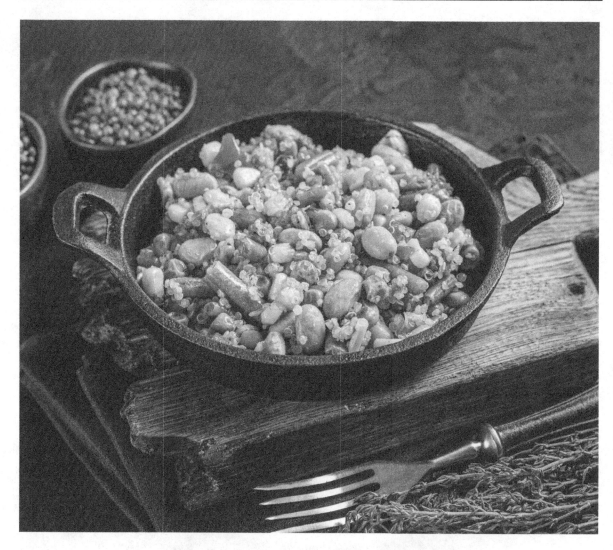

NUTRITIONAL INFORMATION
Calories: 295, Proteins: 7.6g, Carbs: 18.7g, Fat: 22.9g

INGREDIENTS

- 1 c. corn, frozen
- 1/8 tsp. black pepper, grounded
- 2 c. edamame shelled & frozen
- ¼ tsp. chilli powder
- 1 c. quinoa, cooked & cooled
- 1 tbsp. lime juice, fresh
- 1 green onion, sliced
- ¼ tsp. thyme, dried
- 2 tbsps. cilantro, fresh & chopped
- ¼ tsp. salt
- ½ red bell pepper, chopped
- 1 tbsp. lemon juice
- pinch of cayenne pepper
- 1 ½ tbsps. olive oil

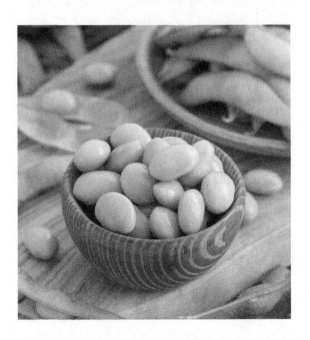

STEP 1
Heat water in a large pot over medium heat.

STEP 2
To this, stir in the edamame and corn.

STEP 3
Boil them slightly and cook them until they are tender.

STEP 4
Once cooked, drain the water and set it aside.

STEP 5
Now, combine all the remaining veggies and quinoa in a large bowl along with the cooked corn and edamame. Toss well.

STEP 6
In the meantime, to make the dressing, mix olive oil, lemon juice, lime juice, black pepper, thyme, chilli powder, and cayenne until emulsified.

STEP 7
Next, drizzle the dressing over the salad and place it in the refrigerator for at least 2 hours. Serve and enjoy.

SIZZLING VEGETARIAN FAJITAS

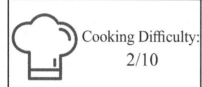 Cooking Difficulty: 2/10	 Cooking Time: 120 minutes	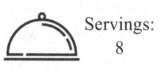 Servings: 8

INGREDIENTS

- 4 oz. diced green chilies
- 3 diced tomatoes
- 1 cored yellow bell pepper, sliced
- 1 cored red bell pepper, sliced
- 1 white onion, peeled and sliced
- ½ tsp. garlic powder
- ¼ tsp. salt
- 2 tsps. red chili powder
- 2 tsps. ground cumin
- ½ tsp. dried oregano
- 1 ½ tbsps. olive oil

STEP 1
Take a 6-quarts slow cooker, grease it with a non-stick cooking spray, and add all the ingredients.

STEP 2
Stir until it mixes properly and cover the top.

STEP 3
Plug in the slow cooker; adjust the cooking time to 2 hours and let it cook on the high heat setting or until cooks thoroughly.

STEP 4
Serve with tortillas.

NUTRITIONAL INFORMATION
Calories:220 Cal, Carbs:73g, Protein:12g, Fats:8g

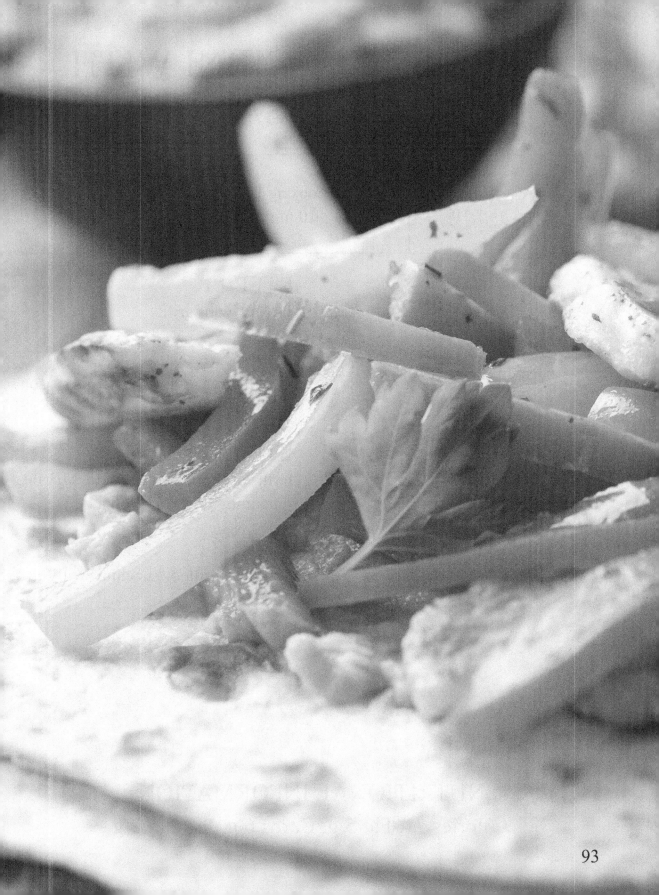

GRILLED ZUCCHINI WITH TOMATO SALSA

 Cooking Difficulty: 3/10

 Cooking Time: 10 minutes

 Servings: 2

INGREDIENTS

- 2 zucchinis, sliced
- 1 tbsp. olive oil
- salt and pepper
- 1 c. tomatoes, chopped
- 1 tbsp. mint, chopped
- 1 tsp. red wine vinegar

STEP 1
Preheat your grill.

STEP 2
Coat the zucchini with oil and season with salt and pepper.

STEP 3
Grill for 4 minutes per side. Mix the remaining ingredients in a bowl.

STEP 4
Top the grilled zucchini with the minty salsa.

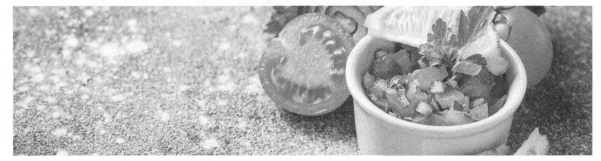

NUTRITIONAL INFORMATION
Calories 71, Fat 5 g, Carbs 6 g, Protein 2 g

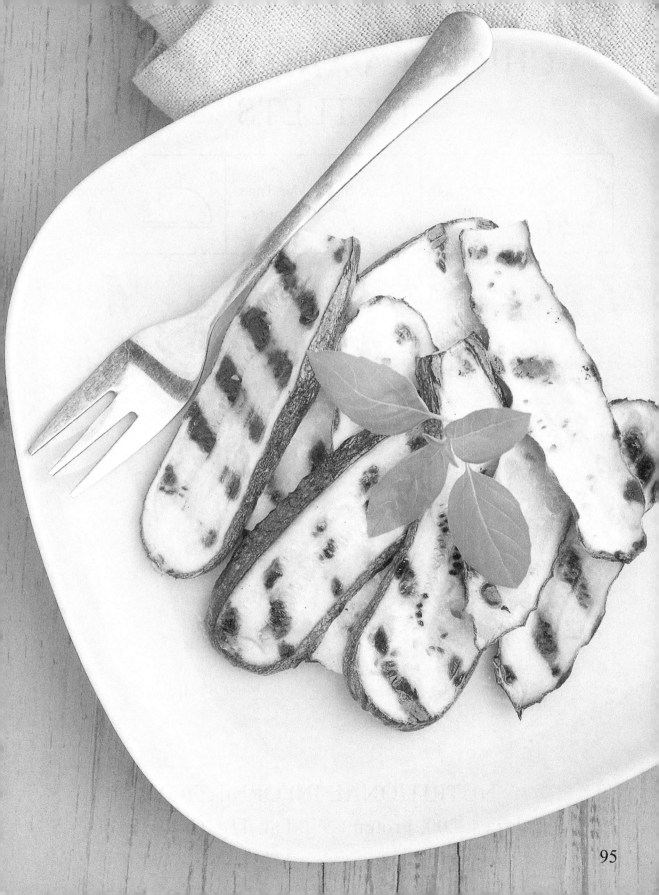

CHICKPEA AND SPINACH CUTLETS

Cooking Difficulty: 3/10	Cooking Time: 40 minutes	Servings: 12

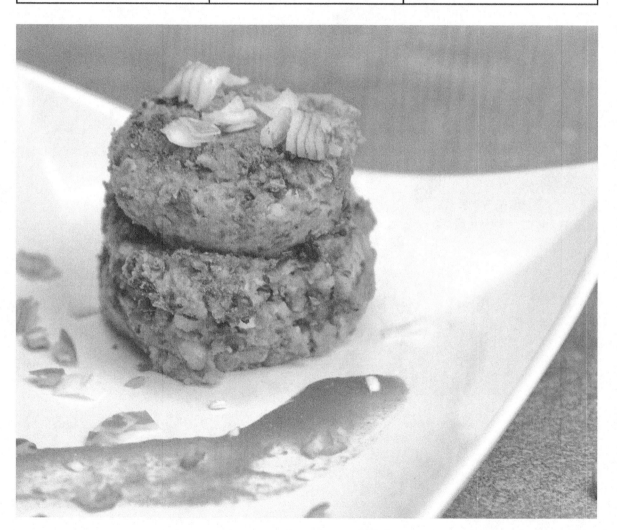

NUTRITIONAL INFORMATION
Calories: 200, Protein: 8 g, Fat: 11g, Carbs: 21 g

INGREDIENTS

- 1 red bell pepper
- 19 oz. chickpeas, rinsed & drained
- 1 c. ground almonds
- 2 tsps. dijon mustard
- 1 tsp. oregano
- ½ tsp. sage
- 1 c. spinach, fresh
- 1½ c. rolled oats
- 1 clove garlic, pressed
- ½ lemon, juiced
- 2 tsps. maple syrup, pure

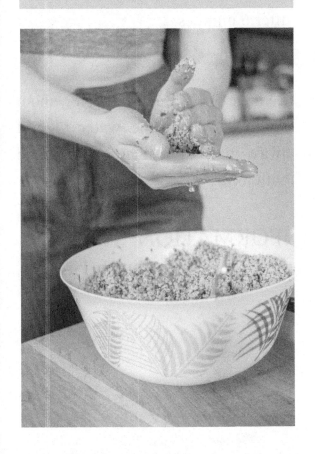

STEP 1
Get out a baking sheet. Line it with parchment paper.

STEP 2
Cut your red pepper in half and then take the seeds out. Place it on your baking sheet, and roast in the oven while you prepare your other ingredients.

STEP 3
Process your chickpeas, almonds, mustard, and maple syrup together in a food processor.

STEP 4
Add in your lemon juice, oregano, sage, garlic, and spinach, processing again. Make sure it's combined, but don't puree it.

STEP 5
Once your red bell pepper is softened, which should roughly take ten minutes, add this to the processor as well. Add in your oats, mixing well.

STEP 6
Form twelve patties, cooking in the oven for a half hour. They should be browned.

PASTA WITH BROCCOLI

 Cooking Difficulty: 3/10

 Cooking Time: 20 minutes

 Servings: 4

INGREDIENTS

- 2 cups durum wheat pasta
- 1 tbsp. garlic
- 1/4 tsp salt
- 1 tbsp. lemon juice
- 2.5 cups water
- 1 cup broccoli
- 2 tbsp. olive oil

STEP 1

Heat oil in a deep frying pan, add garlic, fry lemon juice for about 3 minutes. Add pasta, cover with water and mix well. Bring to a boil, reduce heat and cook until al dente for about 11 minutes; add chopped broccoli after 6 minutes.

STEP 2

Remove the lid and cook for about 3-4 minutes for the water to boil away. Place on a plate and sprinkle with tofu.

NUTRITIONAL INFORMATION
Calories: 211, Fat: 2.4 g, Carbs: 11.2g, Protein: 6.1g

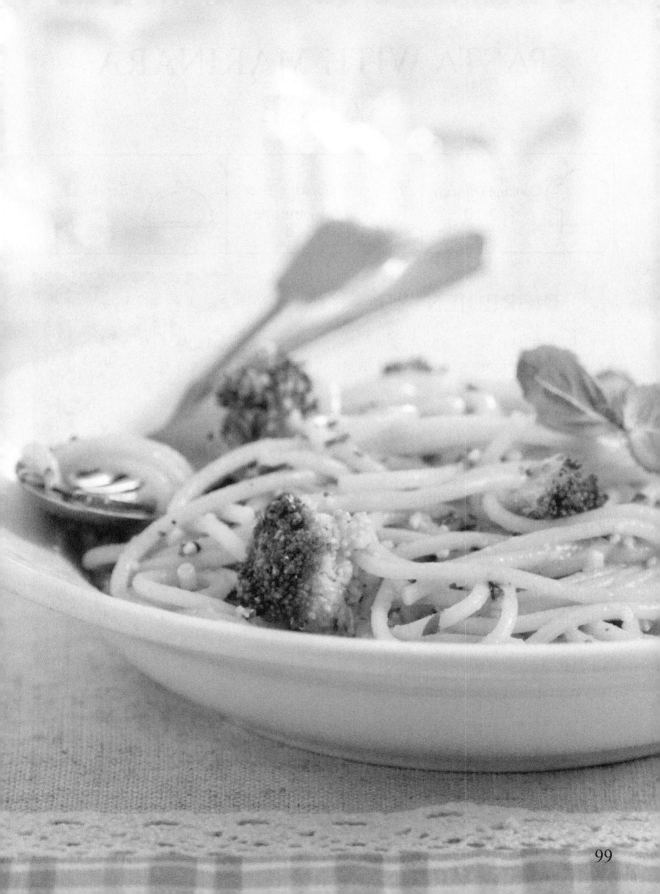

PASTA WITH MARINARA SAUCE

Cooking Difficulty: 2/10	Cooking Time: 14 minutes	Servings: 2

INGREDIENTS

- 4 oz. pasta
- 1 cup marinara sauce
- salt
- hummus

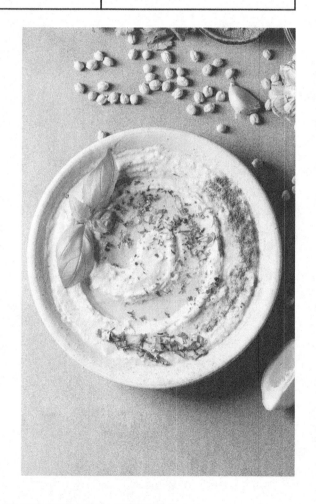

STEP 1
Boil the pasta according to the packaging instructions.

STEP 2
Combine the prepared pasta with the sauce and salt.

STEP 3
Serve the pasta with hummus.

NUTRITIONAL INFORMATION
Calories 360, Fat 3.7g, Carbs 2.1g, Protein 3.7g

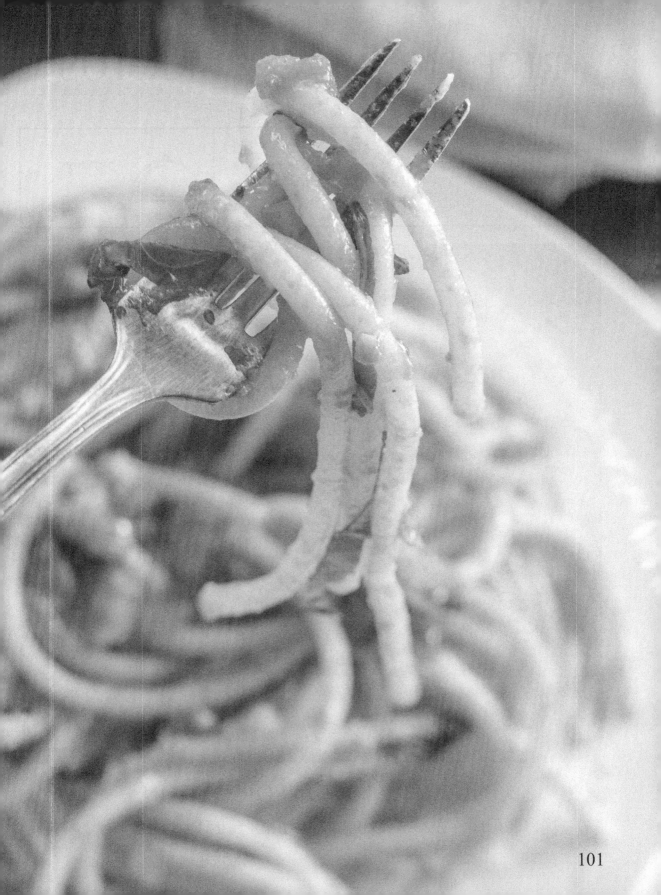

RICE AND BEAN BURRITOS

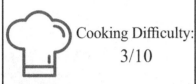 Cooking Difficulty: 3/10	Cooking Time: 20 minutes	Servings: 8

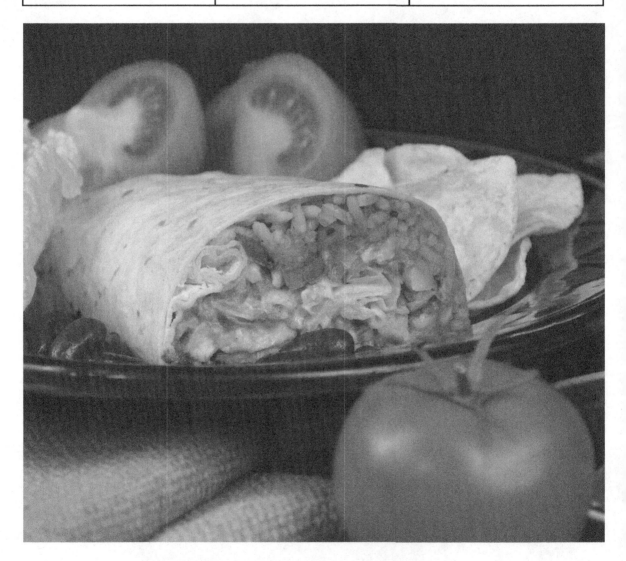

NUTRITIONAL INFORMATION
Calories 290, Carbs 49 g, Fats 6 g, Protein 9 g

INGREDIENTS

- 32 oz. fat-free refried beans
- 6 tortillas
- 2 c. cooked rice
- ½ c. salsa
- 1 tbsp. olive oil
- 1 bunch green onions, chopped
- 2 bell peppers, chopped
- guacamole

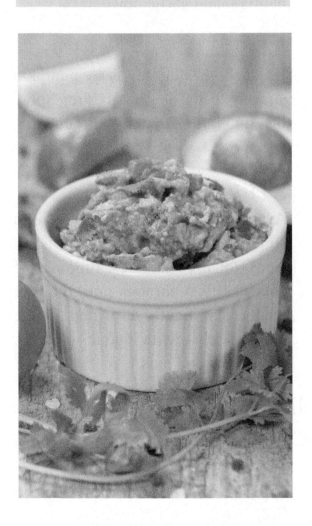

STEP 1
Preheat the oven to 375°F.

STEP 2
Dump the refried beans into a saucepan and place over medium heat to warm.

STEP 3
Heat the tortillas and lay them out on a flat surface.

STEP 4
Spoon the beans in a long mound that runs across the tortilla, just a little off from center.

STEP 5
Spoon some rice and salsa over the beans; add the green pepper and onions to taste, along with any other finely chopped vegetables you like.

STEP 6
Fold over the shortest edge of the plain tortilla and roll it up, folding in the sides as you go.

STEP 7
Place each burrito, seam side down, on a nonstick-sprayed baking sheet.

STEP 8
Brush with olive oil and bake for 15 minutes. Serve with guacamole.

AIR FRYER PUMPKIN SLICES

 Cooking Difficulty: 1/10	 Cooking Time: 12 minutes	 Servings: 4

INGREDIENTS

- 1 medium pumpkin, sliced into 1/2 inch rounds
- 2 tablespoons olive oil
- 1 teaspoon salt
- 1/2 teaspoon black pepper
- 1/2 teaspoon paprika
- 1/4 teaspoon garlic powder
- Cooking spray

STEP 1
Preheat the air fryer to 375°F for 5 minutes. In a mixing bowl, combine the olive oil, salt, black pepper, paprika, and garlic powder.

STEP 2
Brush both sides of each pumpkin slice with the spice mixture. Spray the air fryer basket with cooking spray.

STEP 3
Arrange the pumpkin slices in a single layer in the air fryer basket. Cook for 8-10 minutes, flipping the slices halfway through until they are tender and lightly browned. Serve immediately with your favorite vegetables and nuts.

NUTRITIONAL INFORMATION
Calories 73, Fat 5g, Carbs 7g, Protein 1g

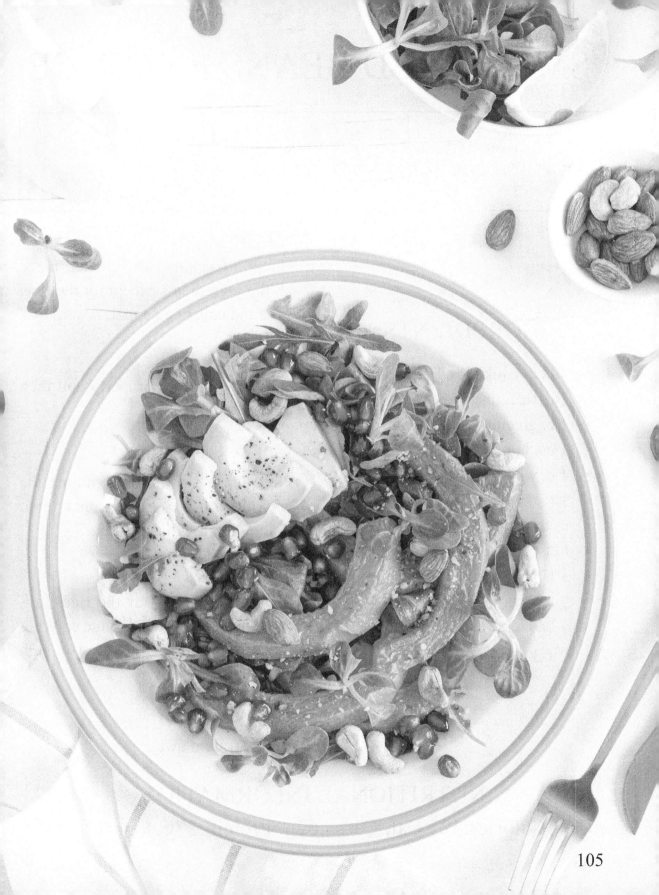

SMOKY RED BEANS AND RICE

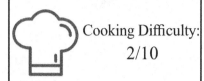 Cooking Difficulty:
2/10

 Cooking Time:
365 minutes

 Servings:
6

INGREDIENTS

- 30 oz. cooked red beans
- 1 c. rice, uncooked
- 1 c. green pepper, chopped
- 1 c. chopped celery
- 1 c. white onion, chopped
- 1 ½ tsps. minced garlic
- ½ tsp. salt
- ¼ tsp. cayenne pepper
- 1 tsp. smoked paprika
- 2 tsps. dried thyme
- 1 bay leaf
- 2 1/3 c. vegetable broth

STEP 1
Using a 6-quarts slow cooker, place all the ingredients except for the rice, salt, and cayenne pepper.

STEP 2
Stir until it mixes properly and then cover the top.

STEP 3
Plug in the slow cooker; adjust the cooking time to 4 hours and let it steam on a low heat setting.

STEP 4
Then pour in and stir the rice, salt, cayenne pepper and continue cooking for an additional 2 hours at a high heat setting.

STEP 5
Serve straight away.

NUTRITIONAL INFORMATION
Calories:425 Cal, Carbs:62g, Protein:27g, Fats:22g

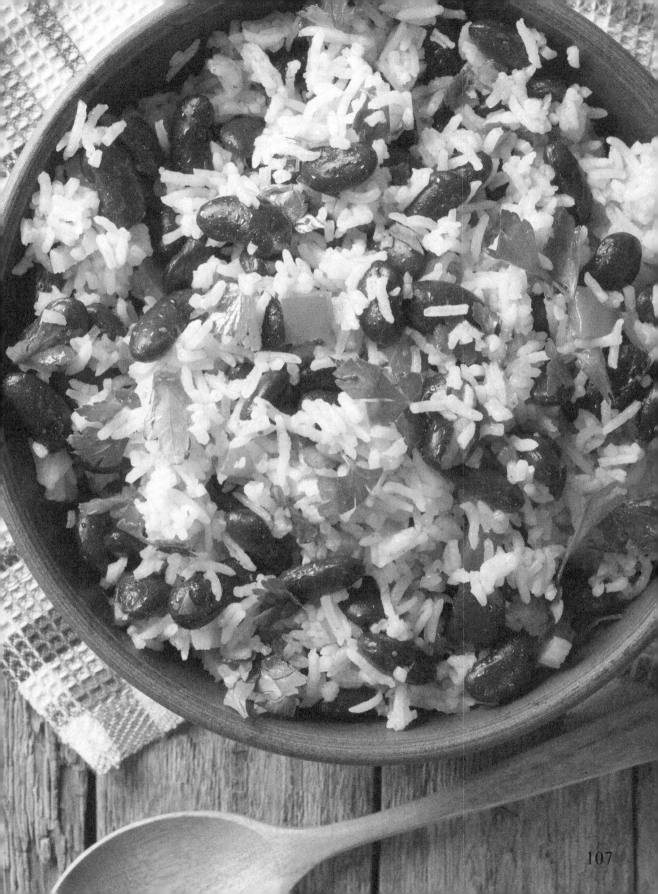

CORIANDER SHRIMP SALAD

Cooking Difficulty: 2/10	Cooking Time: 8 minutes	Servings: 4

INGREDIENTS

- 1 tbsp. coriander, chopped
- 1 lb. shrimp, deveined and peeled
- 1 red onion, sliced
- ¼ tsp. black pepper
- 2 c. baby arugula
- 1 tbsp. lemon juice
- 1 tbsp. olive oil
- 1 tbsp. balsamic vinegar

STEP 1

Heat up a pan with the oil over medium heat, add the onion, stir and sauté for 2 minutes.

STEP 2

Add the shrimp and the other ingredients, toss, cook for 6 minutes, divide into bowls and serve for lunch.

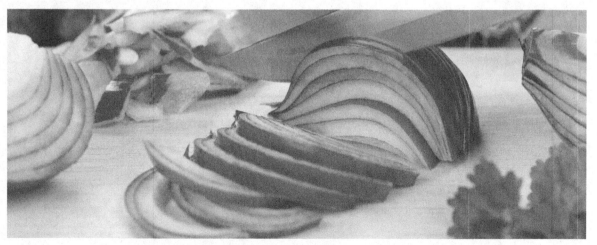

NUTRITIONAL INFORMATION
Calories 341, Fat 11.5g, Carbs 17.3g, Protein 14.3g

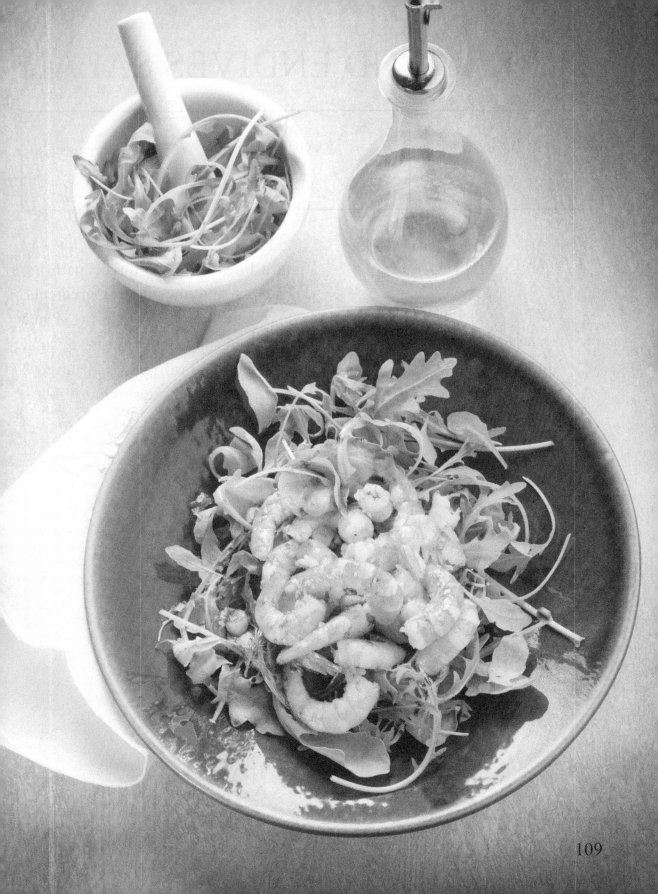

TURKEY AND ENDIVES SALAD

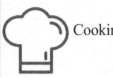 Cooking Difficulty: 1/10

 Cooking Time: 2 minutes

 Servings: 4

INGREDIENTS

- 1 sliced cooked turkey breast, skinless and boneless
- 2 tbsps. avocado oil
- 2 shredded endives
- 1 c. halved cherry tomatoes
- 2 tbsps. lime juice
- 2 tbsps. balsamic vinegar
- 2 tbsps. chopped chives
- black pepper

STEP 1

In a bowl, mix the turkey with the endives and the other ingredients, toss and serve for lunch. Place remaining portions in an airtight container and refrigerate for up to 2 days. Reheat before serving.

NUTRITIONAL INFORMATION
Calories 200, Fat 10g, Carbs 3g, Protein 7g

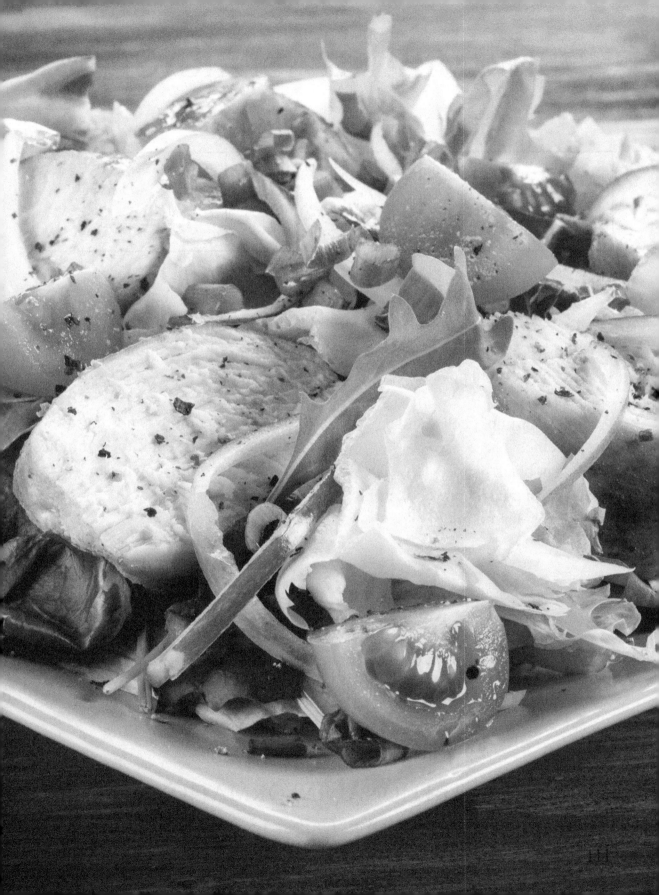

SHRIMP AND ASPARAGUS SALAD

Cooking Difficulty: 2/10	Cooking Time: 12 minutes	Servings: 4

INGREDIENTS

- ¼ c. raspberry vinegar
- 2 tbsps. olive oil
- 2 c. cherry tomatoes halved (optional)
- 2 lbs. shrimp, peeled and deveined
- ¼ tsp. black pepper
- 1 lb. asparagus, pre-cooked
- 1 tbsps. lemon juice

STEP 1

Heat up a pan with the oil over medium-high heat, add the shrimp, toss and cook for 2 minutes.

STEP 2

Add the asparagus and the other ingredients, toss, cook for 8 minutes more, divide into bowls, and serve for lunch.

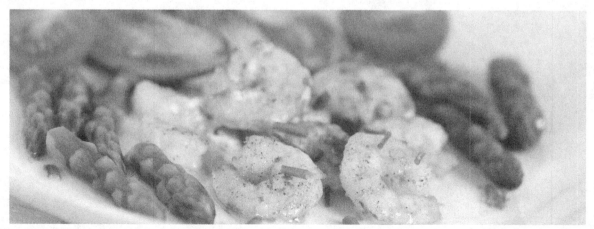

NUTRITIONAL INFORMATION
Calories: 79, Fat: 0.4 g, Carbs: 15 g, Protein: 1.3 g

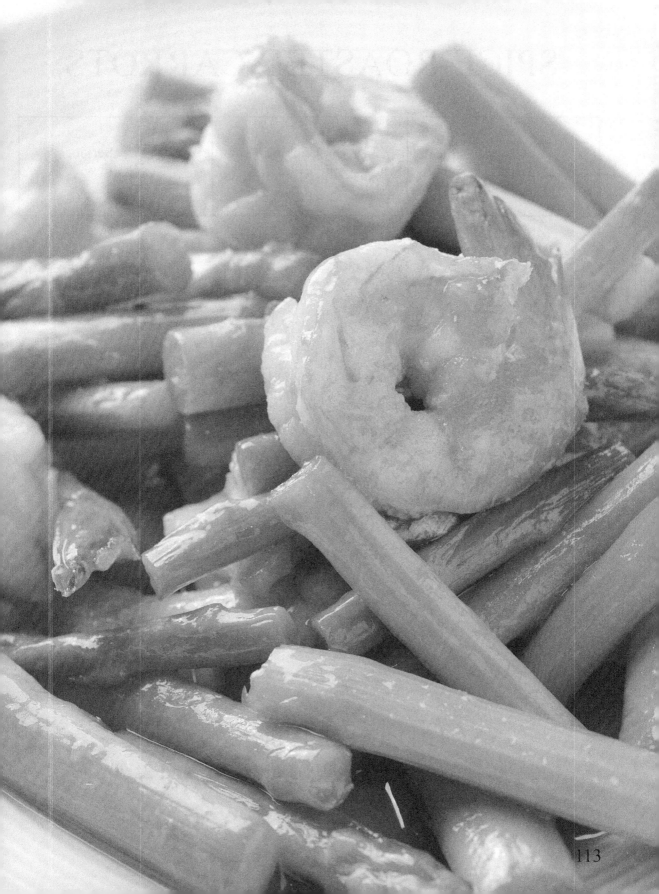

SPICE-ROASTED CARROTS

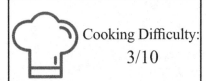 Cooking Difficulty: 3/10	Cooking Time: 55 minutes	Servings: 2

INGREDIENTS

- 8 large carrots
- 3 tbsps. olive oil
- 1 tbsp. red wine vinegar
- 2 tbsps. packed fresh oregano leaves
- 1 tsp. smoked paprika
- ½ tsp. ground nutmeg
- 1 tbsps. vegan butter
- ⅓ c. salted pistachios, roasted
- salt and pepper

STEP 1
Set your oven to 450 degrees F.

STEP 2
Mix oregano, oil, nutmeg, paprika, carrots, salt, and pepper in a roasting pan.

STEP 3
Roast the mixture for about an hour or until carrots become tender.

STEP 4
Transfer to a plate.

STEP 5
Top with vinegar, butter, and top with pistachios before serving.

NUTRITIONAL INFORMATION
120 Calories, 3.5g Fats, 20g Net Carbs, and 2g Protein

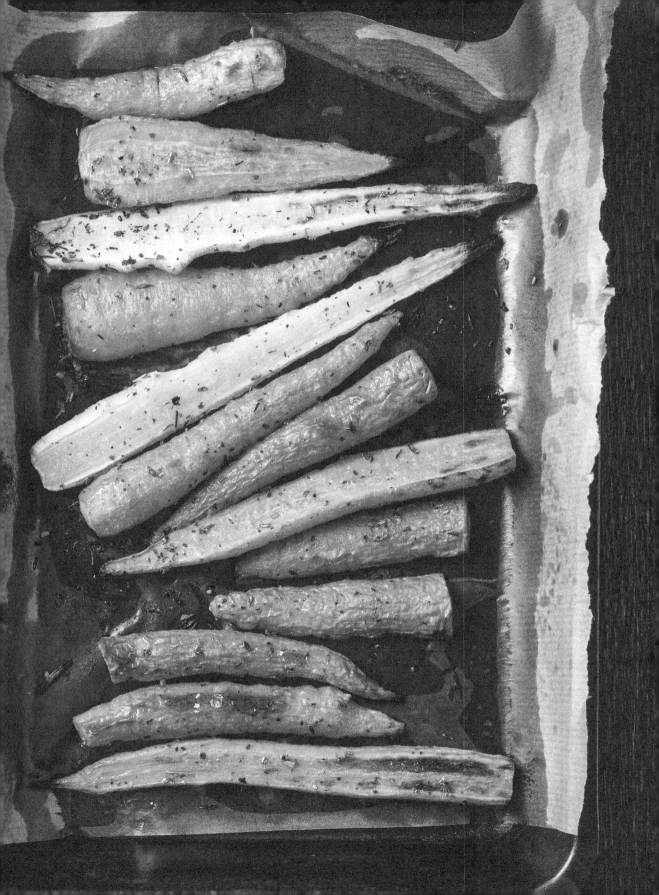

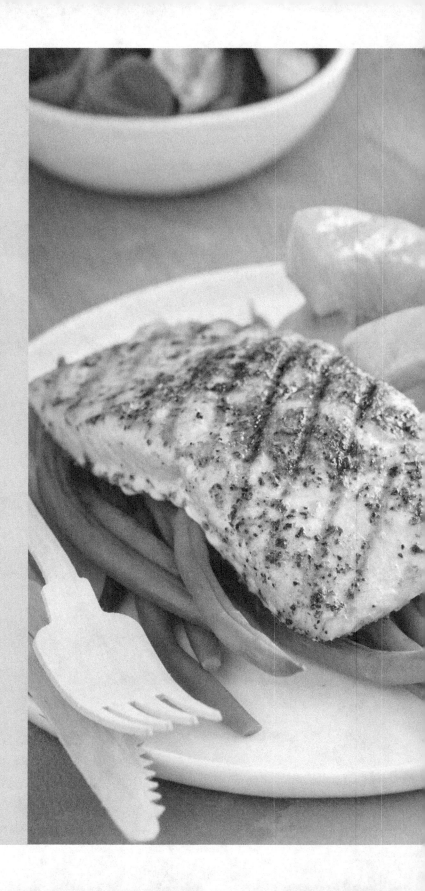

DINNER RECIPES

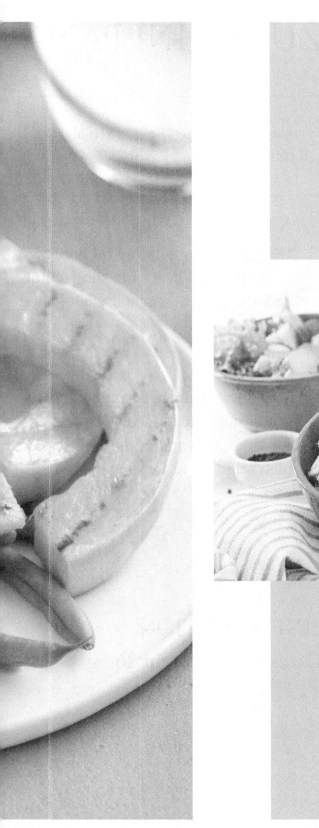
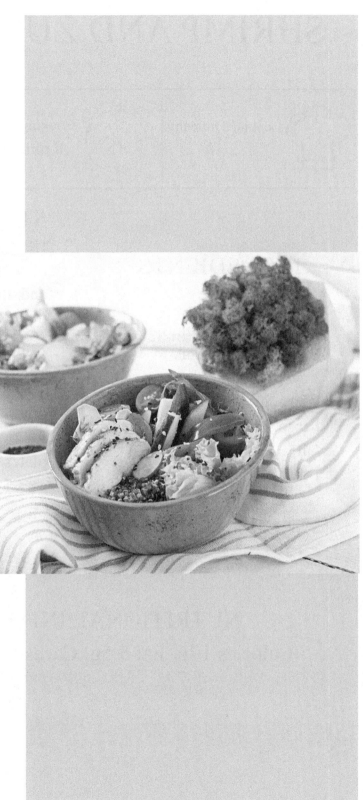

SHRIMP AND ZUCCHINI PAN

 Cooking Difficulty: 2/10

 Cooking Time: 8 minutes

 Servings: 4

INGREDIENTS

- 1 tbsp. olive oil
- 1 lb. deveined shrimp, peeled
- 1 c. sliced zucchinis
- 2 chopped shallots
- 1 tbsp. granulated garlic
- 1 tbsp. red chili flakes
- salt
- 1 tbsp. chopped basil

STEP 1

Heat up a pan with the oil and ghee over medium heat; add the shallots and the garlic, stir and sauté for 2 minutes.

STEP 2

Add the shrimp, zucchinis, and the other ingredients, cook everything for 6 minutes more, divide between plates and serve for dinner.

NUTRITIONAL INFORMATION

Calories 176, Fat 5.5g, Carbs 4.2g, Protein 26.5g

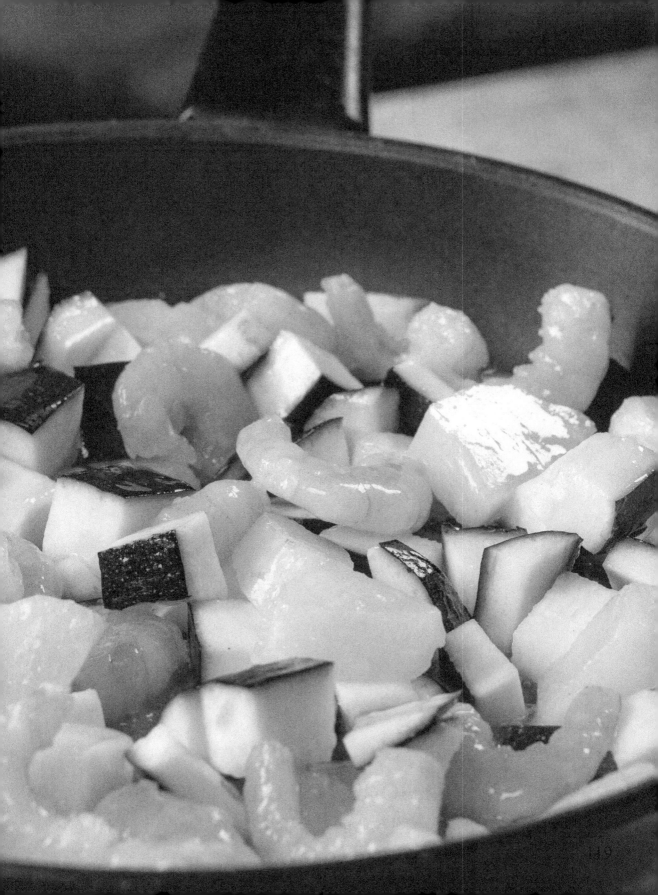

BLACK BEAN STUFFED SWEET POTATOES

Cooking Difficulty: 4/10	Cooking Time: 80 minutes	Servings: 4

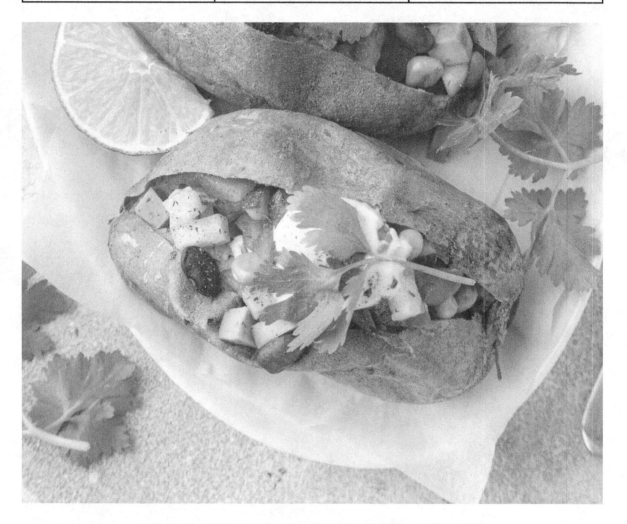

NUTRITIONAL INFORMATION
Calories: 387, Fat: 16.1 g, Carbs: 53 g, Protein: 10.4 g

INGREDIENTS

- 4 sweet potatoes
- 15 oz. cooked black beans
- ½ tsp. ground black pepper
- ½ red onion, peeled, diced
- ½ tsp. sea salt
- ¼ tsp. onion powder
- ¼ tsp. garlic powder
- ¼ tsp. red chili powder
- ¼ tsp. cumin
- 1 tsp. lime juice
- 1 ½ tbsps. olive oil
- ½ c. cashew cream sauce

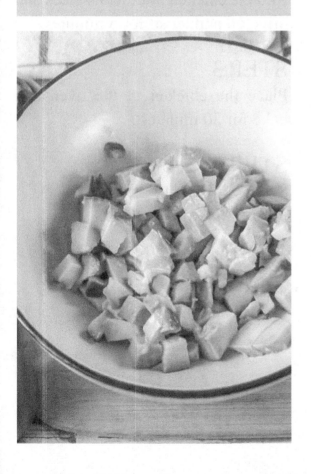

STEP 1
Spread sweet potatoes on a baking tray greased with oil and bake for 65 minutes at 350 degrees f until tender.

STEP 2
Meanwhile, prepare the sauce, and for this, whisk together the cream sauce, black pepper, and lime juice until combined, set aside until required.

STEP 3
When 10 minutes of the baking time of potatoes are left, heat a skillet pan with oil. Add in onion to cook until golden for 5 minutes.

STEP 4
Then stir in spice, cook for another 3 minutes, stir in bean until combined and cook for 5 minutes until hot.

STEP 5
Let roasted sweet potatoes cool for 10 minutes, then cut them open, mash the flesh and top with bean mixture, cilantro and avocado, and then drizzle with cream sauce.

STEP 6
Serve straight away.

BAKED CHICKEN WITH SWEET PAPRIKA

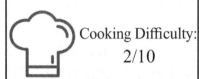 Cooking Difficulty: 2/10

 Cooking Time: 35 minutes

 Servings: 2

INGREDIENTS

- 2 chicken fillets
- 1 tbsp. sweet paprika
- 2 tbsp. olive oil
- 1 tbsp. dried garlic
- salt
- black pepper

STEP 1
Preheat oven to 360 F.

STEP 2
Rub the chicken fillet with spices and olive oil and let sit for 5 minutes.

STEP 3
Place the chicken in the oven and bake for 30 minutes.

STEP 4
Serve with salad.

NUTRITIONAL INFORMATION
Calories 298, Fat 9,3g, Carbs 6g, Protein 11g

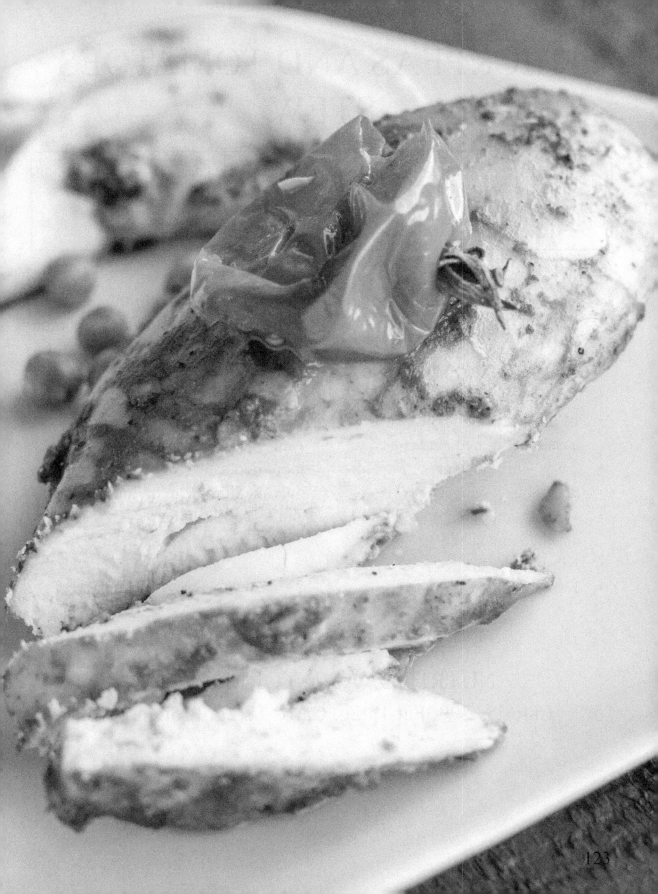

CHICKPEAS AND TOMATOES STEW

Cooking Difficulty: 3/10	Cooking Time: 22 minutes	Servings: 4

INGREDIENTS

- 1 c. low-sodium chicken stock
- 1 yellow onion, chopped
- 14 oz. canned chickpeas, unsalted, drained, and rinsed
- 2 tsps. chili powder
- ¼ tsp. black pepper
- 14 oz. canned tomatoes, unsalted and cubed
- 1 tbsp. olive oil
- 1 tbsp. cilantro, chopped

STEP 1

Heat up a pot with the oil over medium-high heat, add the onion and chili powder, stir and cook for 5 minutes.

STEP 2

Add the chickpeas and the other ingredients, toss, cook for 15 minutes over medium heat, divide into bowls and serve for dinner.

NUTRITIONAL INFORMATION

Calories 299, Fat 13.2g, Carbs 17.2g, Protein 8.1g

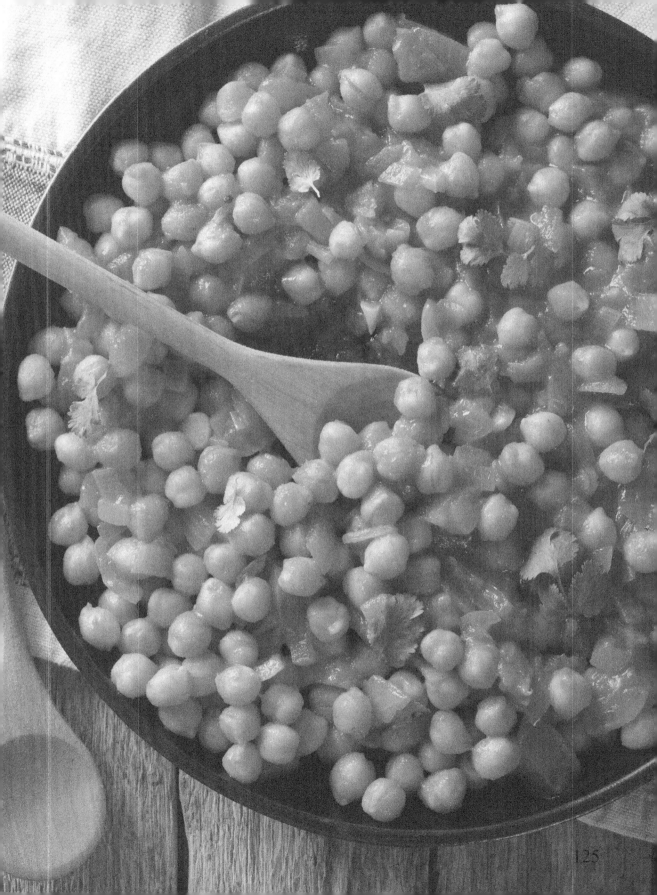

CHICKEN PIECES

 Cooking Difficulty: 3/10	Cooking Time: 15 minutes	Servings: 6

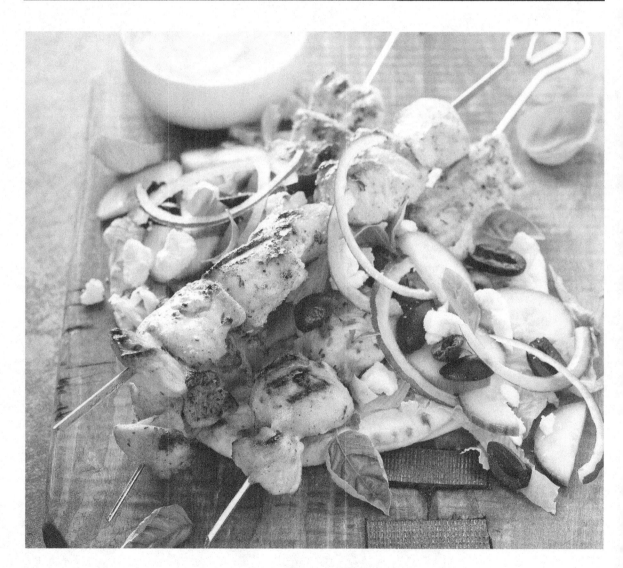

NUTRITIONAL INFORMATION
294 Calories, 5.2g Fat, 42.1g Carbs, 22.2g Protein

INGREDIENTS

- 2 tbsps. lime juice
- 14 oz. Greek yogurt
- 2 tsps. oregano
- ¼ c. white dry wine
- ¼ c. olive oil
- ½ tsp. pepper
- 1 tsp. kosher salt
- 2 lb. skinned breasts
- 1 tsp. granulated garlic
- 2 tsps. distilled white vinegar
- ½ c. cucumber

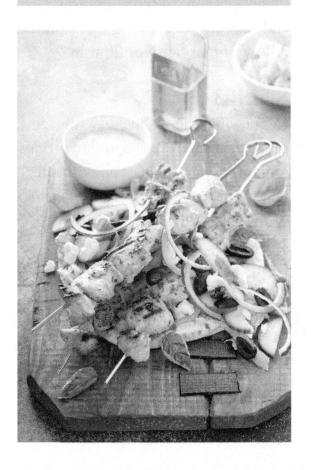

STEP 1

Cut the chicken into ½-inch cubes, and coarsely shred the cucumber.

STEP 2

Set the grill between 450ºF and 550ºF.

STEP 3

Blend the wine, oil, chicken, oregano, lime juice, ¼ teaspoon of the pepper, and the salt in a mixing bowl.

STEP 4

Use eight metal skewers to prepare the chicken for cooking. Grill for approximately 10-12 minutes.

STEP 5

Remove any excess moisture from the cucumbers with paper towels, and put them into a medium dish. Mix in the yogurt, garlic, vinegar, and pepper with the cucumbers.

STEP 6

Serve with warm pita bread and the chicken. Place remaining portions in an airtight container and refrigerate for up to 4 days. Reheat before serving.

SALMON TERIYAKI

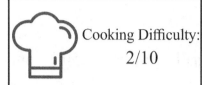 Cooking Difficulty: 2/10	Cooking Time: 27 minutes	Servings: 4

INGREDIENTS

- 6 tbsp. soy sauce
- 2 tbsp. chopped fresh ginger
- 2 tsp. minced garlic
- 4 salmon filet
- 2 tbsp. sesame seeds
- 1 lemon sliced thin

STEP 1
Whisk together soy sauce ginger and garlic . Add optional sesame seeds if using.

STEP 2
Place salmon files in shallow dish and cover with soy-ginger sauce. Allow to marinate for 20 min.

STEP 3
Cover baking sheet with foil. Place fish on foil and top with any remaining marinade. Top with sliced lemon.

STEP 4
Broil 5-7 min. Serve and enjoy!

NUTRITIONAL INFORMATION
Calories 279, Fat 18.7g, Carbs 9 g, Protein 24.1g

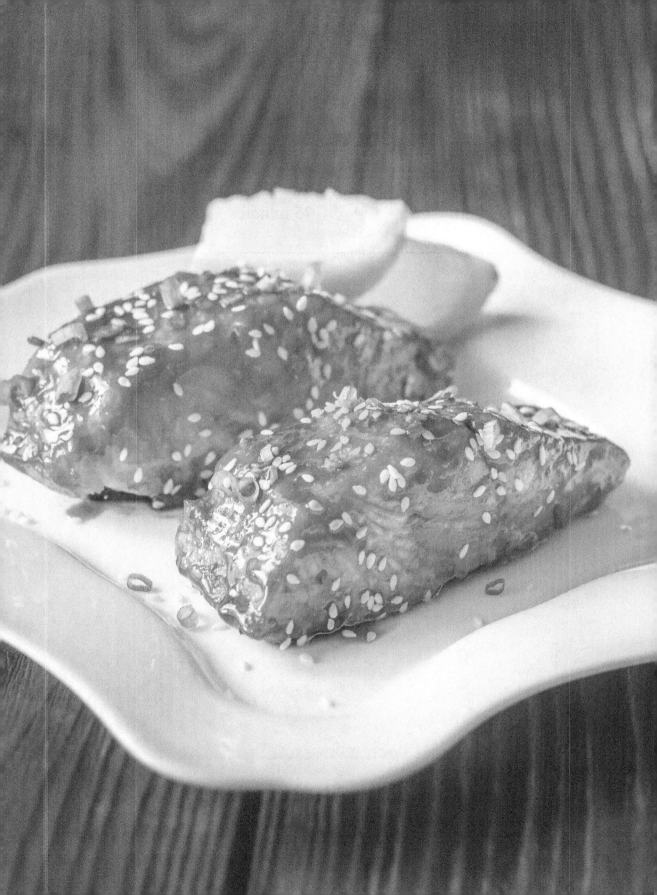

BALSAMIC-GLAZED ROASTED CAULIFLOWER

Cooking Difficulty: 3/10	Cooking Time: 75 minutes	Servings: 4

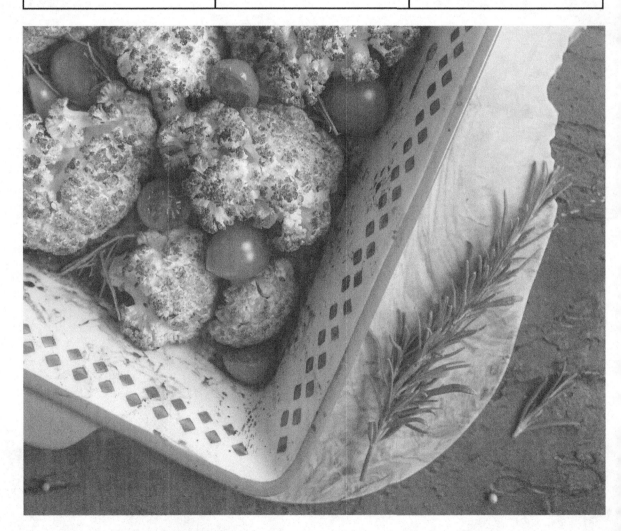

NUTRITIONAL INFORMATION
Calories: 86, Fat: 5.7 g, Carbs: 7.7 g, Protein: 3.1 g

INGREDIENTS

- 1 head cauliflower
- ½ lb. green beans, trimmed
- 1 peeled red onion, wedged
- 2 c. cherry tomatoes
- ½ tsp. salt
- ¼ c. brown sugar
- 3 tbsps. olive oil
- 1 c. balsamic vinegar
- 2 tbsps. chopped parsley, for garnish

STEP 1

Place cauliflower florets in a baking dish, add tomatoes, green beans, and onion wedges around it, season with salt, and drizzle with oil.

STEP 2

Pour vinegar in a saucepan, stir in sugar, bring the mixture to a boil and simmer for 15 minutes until reduced by half.

STEP 3

Brush the sauce generously over cauliflower florets and then roast for 1 hour at 400 degrees f until cooked, brushing sauce frequently.

STEP 4

When done, garnish vegetables with parsley and then serve.

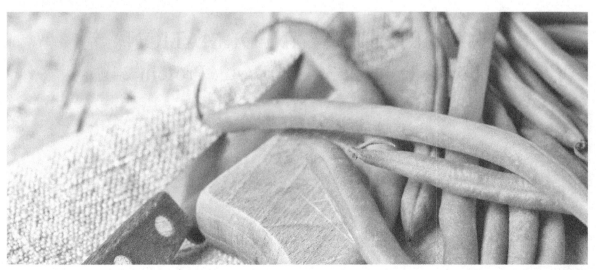

CHILI COD

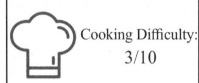 Cooking Difficulty: 3/10	Cooking Time: 8 minutes	Servings: 4

INGREDIENTS

- 4 boneless cod fillets
- 2 tbsps. avocado oil
- salt
- black pepper
- 1 tsp. chili powder
- 1 tbsp. chopped cilantro
- 3 minced garlic cloves
- ½ tsp. crushed chili pepper

STEP 1

Heat up a pan with the oil over medium-high heat, add the garlic, chili pepper, and chili powder, stir then cook for 2 minutes.

STEP 2

Add the fish and the other ingredients, cook for 5 minutes on each side, divide between plates and serve.

NUTRITIONAL INFORMATION

Calories 154, Fat 3g, Carbs 4g, Protein 24g

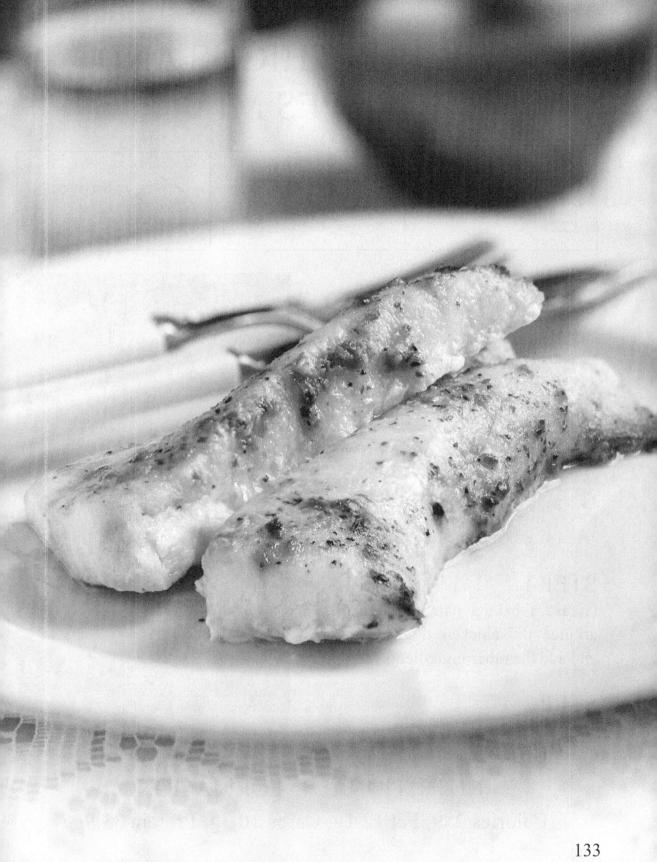

CHICKEN THIGHS AND GRAPES MIX

 Cooking Difficulty: 3/10

 Cooking Time: 42 minutes

 Servings: 4

INGREDIENTS

- 2 garlic cloves, chopped
- 1 c. tomatoes, cubed
- 1 yellow onion, sliced
- black pepper
- ¼ c. chicken stock
- 1 lb. chicken thighs
- 1 carrot, cubed
- 1 tbsp. olive oil
- 1 c. green grapes

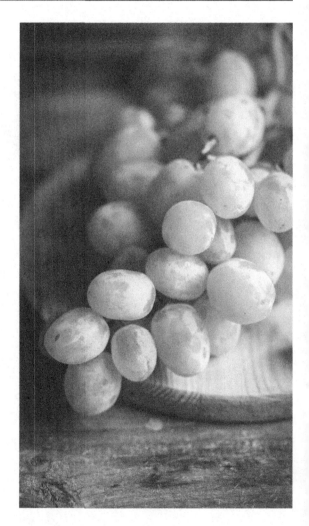

STEP 1
Grease a baking pan with the oil, arrange the chicken thighs inside, and add the other ingredients on top.

STEP 2
Bake at 390 degrees F for 40 minutes, divide between plates and serve.

NUTRITIONAL INFORMATION
Calories 289, Fat 12.1g, Carbs 10.3g, Protein 33.9g

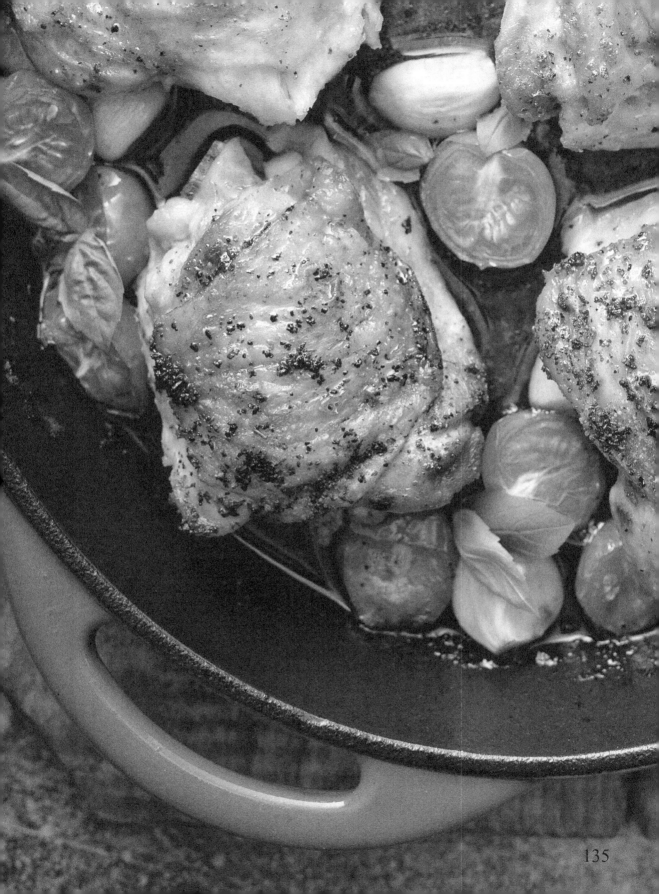

COCONUT CHICKPEA CURRY

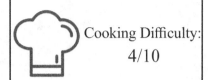 Cooking Difficulty: 4/10	Cooking Time: 27 minutes	Servings: 4

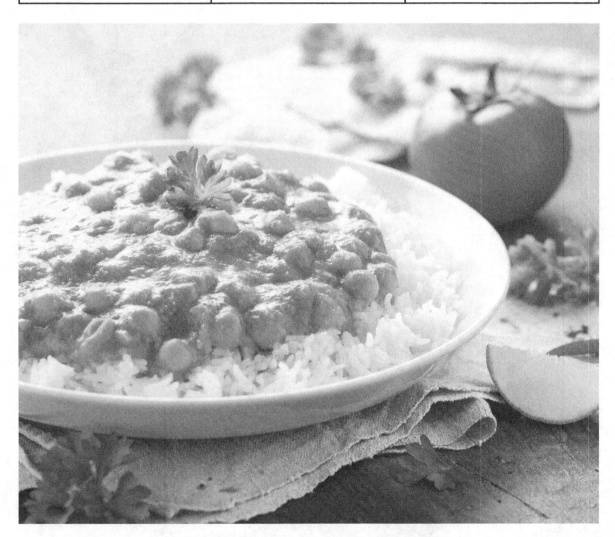

NUTRITIONAL INFORMATION
Calories: 225, Fat: 9.4 g, Carbs: 28.5 g, Protein: 7.3

INGREDIENTS

- 2 tsps. coconut flour
- 16 oz. cooked chickpeas
- 14 oz. tomatoes, diced
- 1 red onion, sliced
- 1 ½ tsps. minced garlic
- ½ tsp. sea salt
- 1 tsp. curry powder
- 1/3 tsp. ground black pepper
- 1 ½ tbsps. garam masala
- ¼ tsp. cumin
- 1 lime, juiced
- 13.5 oz. coconut milk, unsweetened
- 2 tbsps. coconut oil

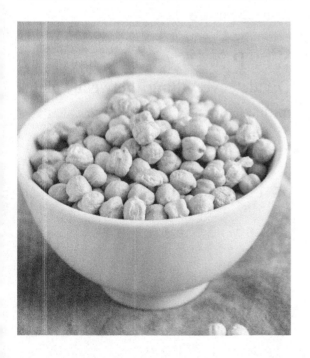

STEP 1
Take a large pot, place it over medium-high heat, add oil and when it melts, add onions and tomatoes, season with salt and black pepper and cook for 5 minutes.

STEP 2
Switch heat to medium-low level, cook for 10 minutes until tomatoes have released their liquid, then add chickpeas and stir in garlic, curry powder, garam masala, and cumin until combined.

STEP 3
Stir in milk and flour, bring the mixture to boil, then switch heat to medium heat and simmer the curry for 12 minutes until cooked.

STEP 4
Taste to adjust seasoning, drizzle with lime juice, and serve. Place remaining portions in an airtight container and refrigerate for up to 2 days. Reheat before serving.

CAULIFLOWER AND TOMATOES MIX

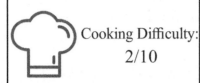 Cooking Difficulty: 2/10	Cooking Time: 30 minutes	Servings: 4

INGREDIENTS

- 1 lb. cauliflower florets
- ½ lb. halved cherry tomatoes
- 2 tbsps. avocado oil
- 2 chopped shallots
- 2 minced garlic cloves
- salt
- black pepper
- 1 c. vegetable stock
- 1 tbsp. chopped coriander
- ½ tsp. ground allspice

STEP 1
Ensure that you heat the pan; add the shallots and the garlic and sauté for 2 minutes.

STEP 2
Add the cauliflower and the other ingredients toss bring to a simmer then cook over medium heat for 28 minutes more.

STEP 3
Divide everything between plates and serve.

NUTRITIONAL INFORMATION
Calories 89, Fat 3.8g, Carbs 13.5g, Protein 2.9g

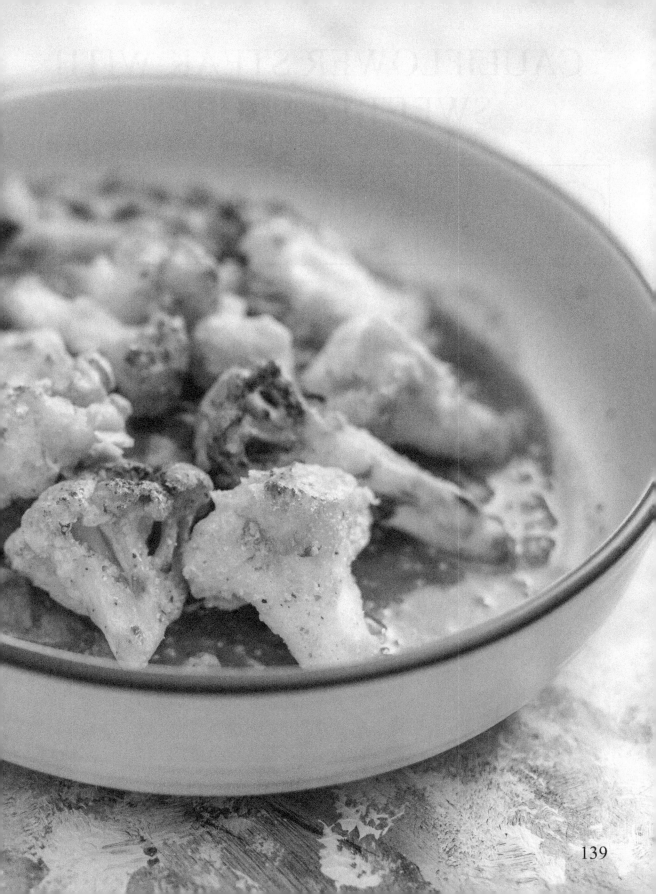

CAULIFLOWER STEAK WITH SWEET-PEA PUREE

 Cooking Difficulty: 3/10

 Cooking Time: 35 minutes

 Servings: 2

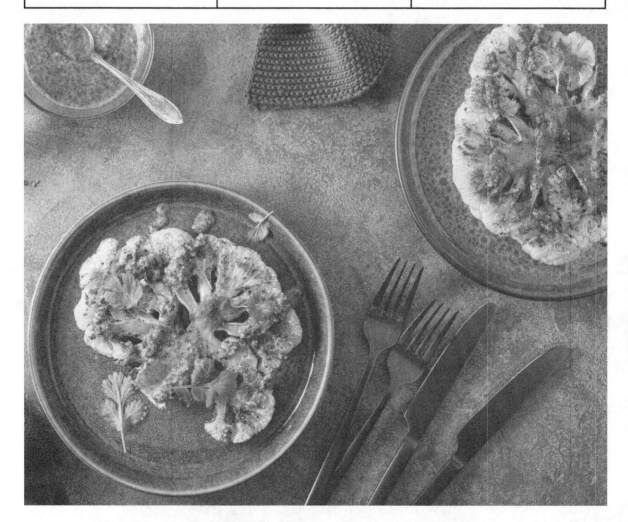

NUTRITIONAL INFORMATION
Calories 234, Fat 3.8g, Carbs 40.3g, Protein 14.5g

INGREDIENTS

cauliflower:
- 2 heads cauliflower
- 1 tsp. olive oil
- ¼ tsp. paprika
- 1 tsp. coriander
- ¼ tsp. black pepper

sweet-pea puree:
- 10 oz. frozen green peas
- 1 onion, chopped
- 2 tbsps. fresh parsley
- ¼ c. unsweetened soy milk

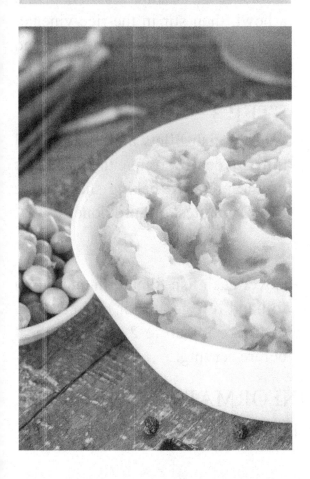

STEP 1
Preheat oven to 425F.

STEP 2
Remove bottom core of cauliflower. Stand it on its base, starting in the middle, slice in half. Then slice steaks about ¾ inches thick.

STEP 3
Using a baking pan, set in the steaks.

STEP 4
Using olive oil, coat the front and back of the steaks.

STEP 5
Sprinkle with coriander, paprika, and pepper.

STEP 6
Bake for 30 minutes, flipping once.

STEP 7
Meanwhile, steam the chopped onion and peas until soft.

STEP 8
Place these vegetables in a blender with milk and parsley and blend until smooth.

GINGER SESAME HALIBUT

Cooking Difficulty: 3/10	Cooking Time: 17 minutes	Servings: 2

INGREDIENTS

- 24 oz. halibut fillets
- 1½ tbsps. minced fresh ginger
- 1½ tsps. soy sauce
- ½ tsps. worcestershire sauce
- 1½ tsps. olive oil
- ¾ tsp. sesame oil
- ¾ tsp. rice wine vinegar

STEP 1
Set the oven to 400 degrees F to preheat. Line a baking sheet with aluminum foil and set aside.

STEP 2
Combine the sesame and olive oils in a bowl, then stir in the rice vinegar, soy sauce, worcestershire sauce and ginger.

STEP 3
Add the fish fillets and turn several times to coat. Arrange the fish fillets on the prepared baking sheet. Bake for 17 minutes, or until done.

STEP 4
Cover each fish fillet with aluminum foil and refrigerate for up to 3 days, or freeze for up to 2 weeks. Reheat before serving.

NUTRITIONAL INFORMATION
237 Calories, 35g Fats, 1g Net Carbs, and 33g Protein

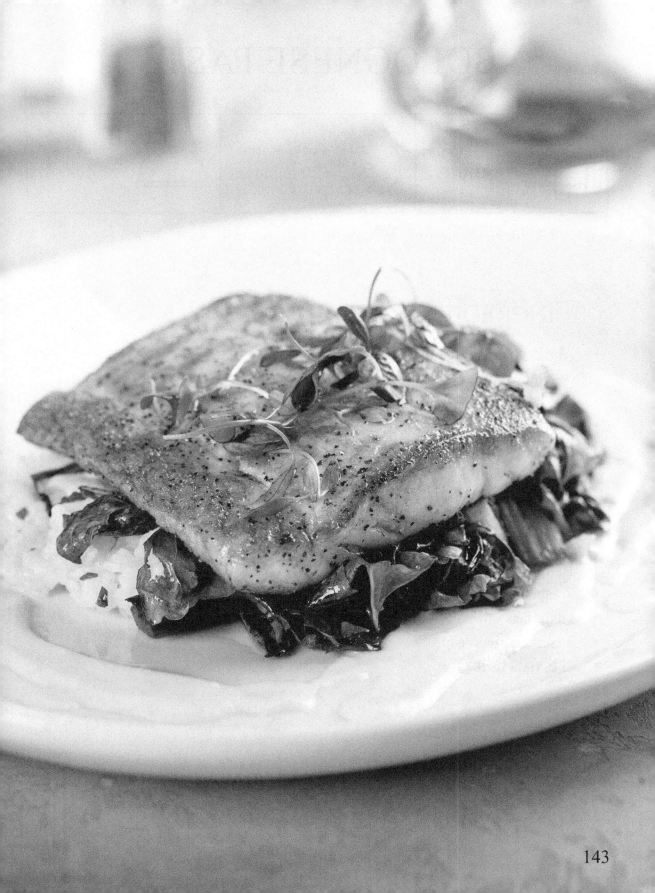

BOLOGNESE PASTA

 Cooking Difficulty: 3/10

 Cooking Time: 20 minutes

 Servings: 4

INGREDIENTS

- 15 oz. garbanzo beans, drained, washed & dried
- ¼ c. extra virgin olive oil
- ¼ c. parsley, fresh & chopped
- 1 carrot, diced
- 24 oz. marinara sauce
- 1 celery stalk, diced
- 4 garlic cloves, minced
- 8 oz. pasta of your choice
- 1 shallot, diced
- ¼ tsp. black pepper, grounded
- 1 tsp. sea salt
- 2 tsp. maple syrup
- ½ c. oats milk

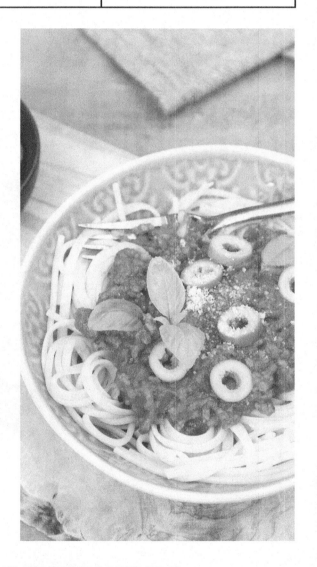

NUTRITIONAL INFORMATION
Calories: 396, Proteins: 22.4g, Carbs: 55.5g, Fat: 11.5g

STEP 1

Heat oil in a large-sized saucepan over medium-high heat.

STEP 2

To this, stir in the carrot, celery, shallots, pepper, and salt.

STEP 3

Now, saute the veggies for 2 to 3 minutes or until softened.

STEP 4

Next, spoon in the garlic and cook for further 1 minute or until aromatic.

STEP 5

Then, place the garbanzo beans in the food processor and process them by pulsing them nine times.

STEP 6

After that, spoon in the processed garbanzo beans and marinara sauce to the saucepan. Mix well.

STEP 7

Once combined, pour the oats milk and maple syrup to it. Combine. Cook for 5 minutes and then lower the heat.

STEP 8

Simmer the mixture for few minutes while keeping it covered with a lid. Meanwhile, boil a pot of water over medium-high heat.

STEP 9

Add the pasta once the water starts boiling and cook by following the manufacturer's instructions. Cook until al dente. Finally, stir in the cooked pasta to the sauce mixture and coat well. Garnish with basil and parsley before serving.

THYME CHICKEN MIX

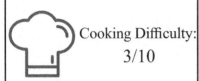 Cooking Difficulty: 3/10

 Cooking Time: 20 minutes

 Servings: 4

INGREDIENTS

- 1 lb. skinless and boneless chicken breast, sliced
- 1 tbsp. olive oil
- 2 chopped spring onions
- 1 c. baby spinach
- 1 tbsp. chopped thyme
- ½ c. tomato passata
- salt
- black pepper

STEP 1

Ensure that you heat the pan, add the spring onions, and the meat and brown for 5 minutes.

STEP 2

Add the rest of the ingredients, bring to a simmer then cook over medium heat for 15 minutes, stirring from time to time.

STEP 3

Divide the mix into bowls and serve.

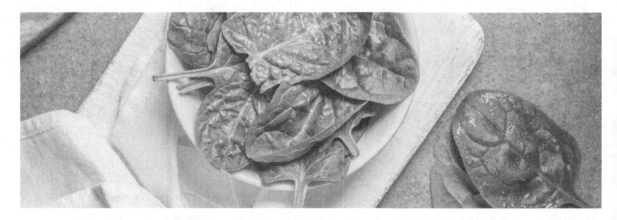

NUTRITIONAL INFORMATION
Calories 380, Fat 40g, Carbs 1g, Protein 17g

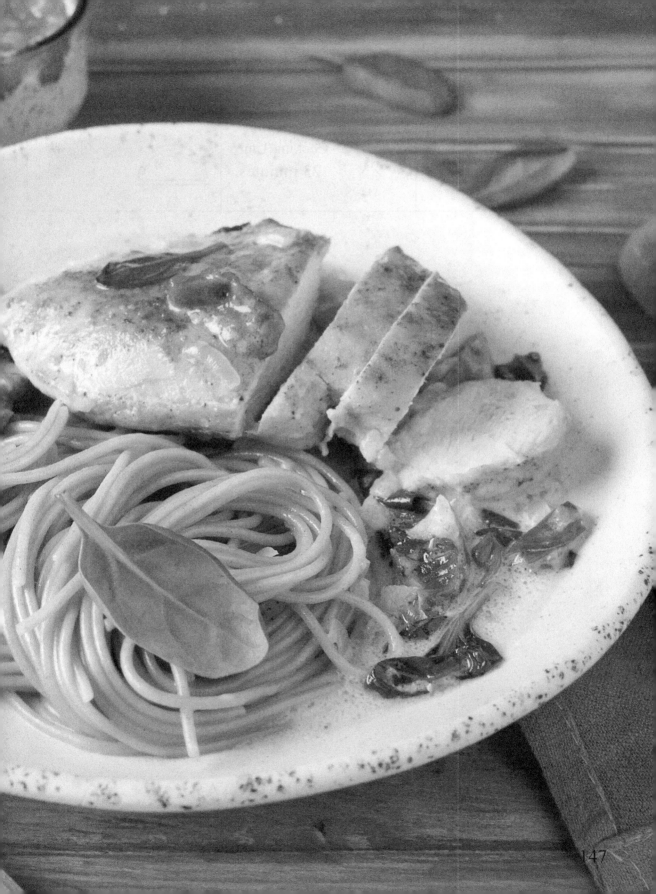

TASTY ROAST SALMON

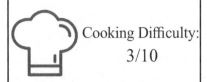 Cooking Difficulty: 3/10	Cooking Time: 23 minutes	Servings: 6

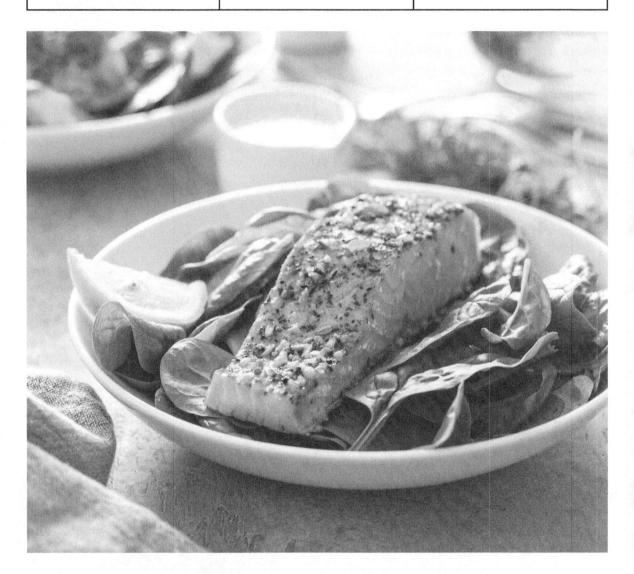

NUTRITIONAL INFORMATION
204.7 Calories, 10.4g Fats, 4.0g Net Carbs, 22.9g Protein

INGREDIENTS

- 1 medium size salmon
- 1 tbsp. olive oil
- 1 tbsp. white wine
- 1 tsp. paprika
- ½ tsp. ground ginger
- ½ tsp. crushed garlic
- 3 tsps. chopped parsley
- 1 lemon, cut into wedges

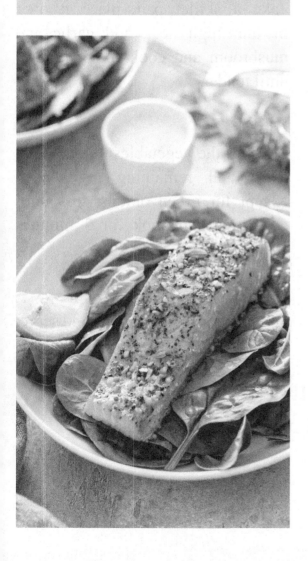

STEP 1

Preheat oven to 400F.

STEP 2

Line a roasting tin with foil, or alternatively simply coat the tin with a little bit of olive oil.

STEP 3

In a good size bowl mix together the garlic, ginger, paprika, chopped parsley and season with salt and pepper. Stir the mix well and then add in the salmon, gently rubbing the marinade over the fish.

STEP 4

Lay the salmon in the prepared tin and top it with a dash of white wine. Roast the fish uncovered for about 20 minutes.

STEP 5

Put the cooked tasty salmon in your serving dish decorated with your choice of herbs and lemon. Make sure pour the remaining juice over the fish.

LINGUINE WITH WILD MUSHROOMS

Cooking Difficulty: 2/10	Cooking Time: 10 minutes	Servings: 4

INGREDIENTS

- 12 oz. mixed mushrooms, sliced
- 2 green onions, sliced
- 1 ½ tsps. minced garlic
- 1 lb. whole-grain linguine pasta, cooked
- ¼ c. nutritional yeast
- ½ tsp. salt
- ¾ tsp. ground black pepper
- 6 tbsps. olive oil
- ¾ c. vegetable stock, hot

STEP 1
Take a skillet pan, place it over medium-high heat, add garlic and mushroom and cook for 5 minutes until tender.

STEP 2
Transfer the vegetables to a pot, add pasta and remaining ingredients, except for green onions, toss until combined and cook for 3 minutes until hot.

STEP 3
Garnish with green onions and serve.

NUTRITIONAL INFORMATION
Calories: 430, Fat: 15 g, Carbs: 62 g, Protein: 15 g

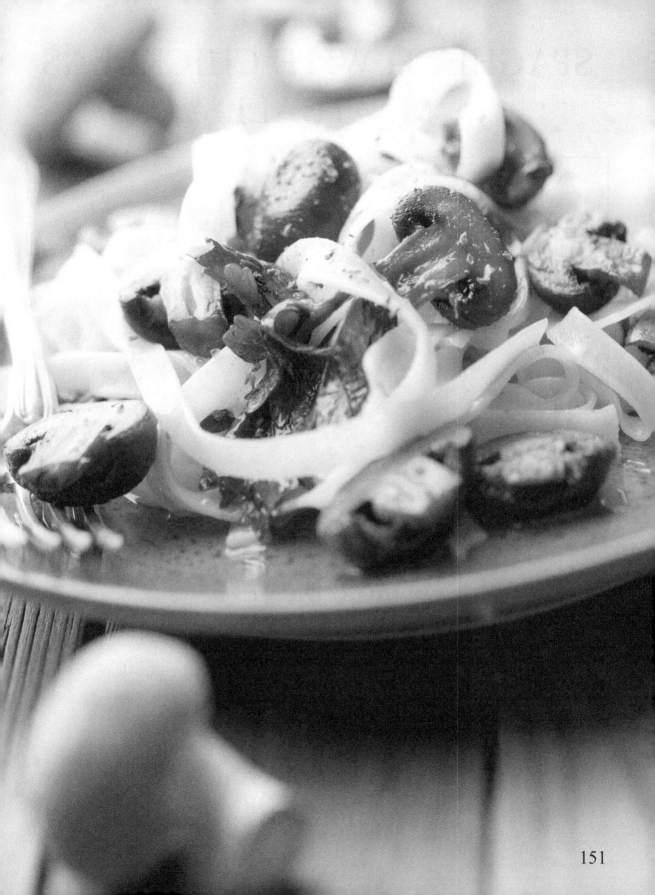

SPAGHETTI WITH CHICKPEAS MEATBALLS

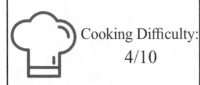 Cooking Difficulty: 4/10

 Cooking Time: 40 minutes

 Servings: 8

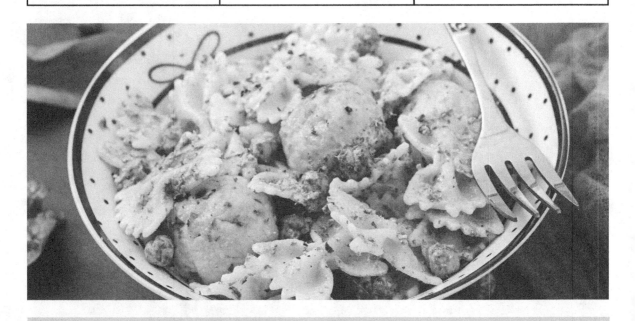

INGREDIENTS

- ½ c. breadcrumbs
- 1 tsp. italian seasoning
- 3 c. chickpeas, drained & rinsed
- ½ tsp. salt
- 3 tbsps. flax seed, grounded
- 2 tsps. onion powder
- 8 tbsps. water
- ½ tbsp. garlic powder
- ¼ c. nutritional yeast
- for the pasta:
- 1 lb. pasta of your choice
- 25 oz. pasta sauce

NUTRITIONAL INFORMATION
Calories: 323, Proteins: 15g, Carbs: 63g, Fat: 4g

STEP 1
First, preheat the oven to 325 °F.

STEP 2
After that, combine the flax seeds with water in a small bowl and set it aside for 5 minutes.

STEP 3
Next, place the chickpeas and salt in the food processor and process them for one minute or until you get a smooth mixture.

STEP 4
Now, transfer the chickpea mixture and the flaxseed mixture to a large mixing bowl. Stir well.

STEP 5
Once combined, add all the remaining ingredients needed to the bowl.

STEP 6
Give everything a good stir and mix well.

STEP 7
Then, make balls out of this mixture and arrange them on a parchment paper-lined baking sheet while leaving ample space in between.

STEP 8
Bake them for 33 to 35 minutes. Turn them once halfway through.

STEP 9
In the meantime, make the pasta by following the instructions given on the packet. Cook until al dente.

STEP 10
Finally, place the spaghetti on the serving plate and top it with the meatballs and pasta sauce. Serve and enjoy.

CASHEW TURKEY MEDLEY

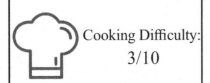 Cooking Difficulty: 3/10	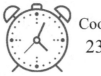 Cooking Time: 23 minutes	Servings: 4

INGREDIENTS

- 1 tbsp. cilantro, chopped
- black pepper
- 1 c. cashews, chopped
- 2 ½ tbsps. cashew butter
- ½ tbsp. olive oil
- ¼ c. chicken stock, low-sodium
- 1 yellow onion, chopped
- 1 lb. turkey breast, skinless, deboned and cubed
- 1 tsp. sweet paprika

STEP 1

Heat up a pan with the oil over medium-high heat, add the onion, stir and sauté for 5 minutes.

STEP 2

Add the meat and brown it for 5 minutes more.

STEP 3

Add the rest of the ingredients, toss, bring to a simmer and cook over medium heat for 30 minutes.

STEP 4

Divide the whole mix between plates and serve.

NUTRITIONAL INFORMATION

Calories 352, Fat 12.7g, Carbs 33.2g, Protein 13.5g

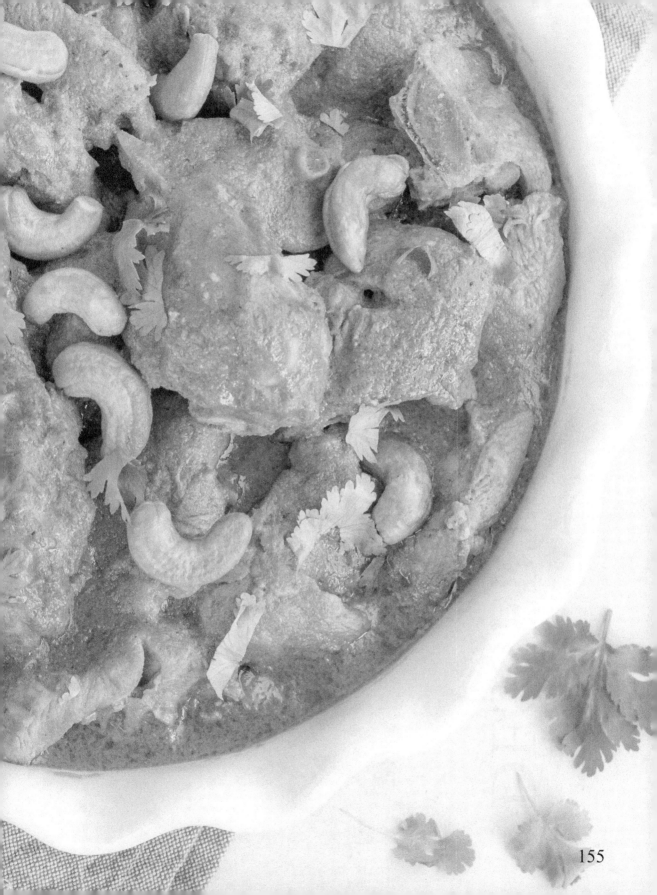

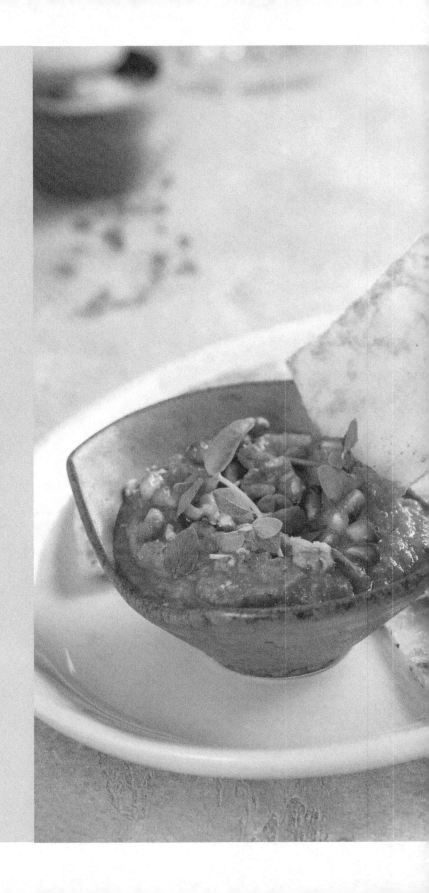

DESSERTS & SNACKS

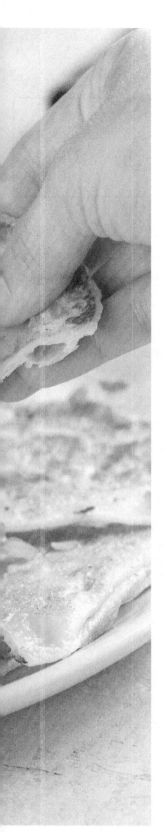

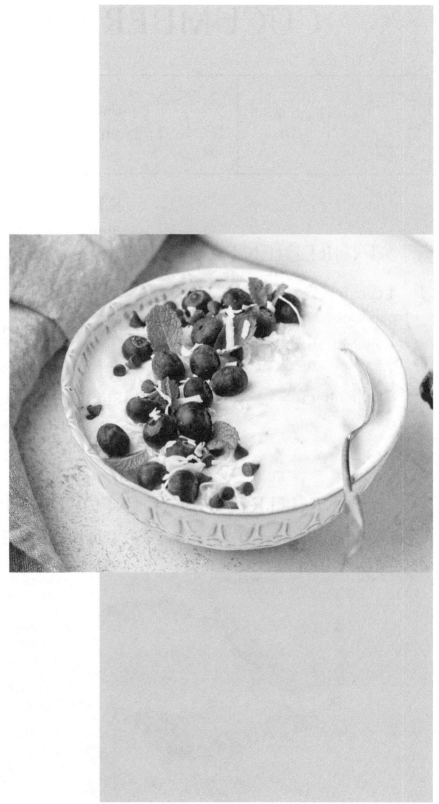

CUCUMBER SALAD

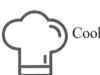 Cooking Difficulty: 2/10	Cooking Time: 25 minutes	Servings: 2

INGREDIENTS

- 4 cucumbers
- parsley
- 1 tsp salt
- 0.5 tbsp. lemon peel
- 1 tsp lemon fresh

STEP 1

Prepare your cucumbers. Cut them into thin strips or rings, put them in a bowl, sprinkle with salt. Add finely chopped parsley. Cover with cling film and refrigerate for 20 minutes.

STEP 2

Stir the cucumbers and put in a salad bowl, season with lemon juice and zest, stir.

NUTRITIONAL INFORMATION

65 Calories, 0,5g Fats, 1g Carbs, and 2g Protein

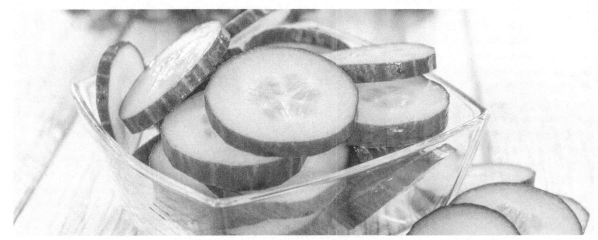

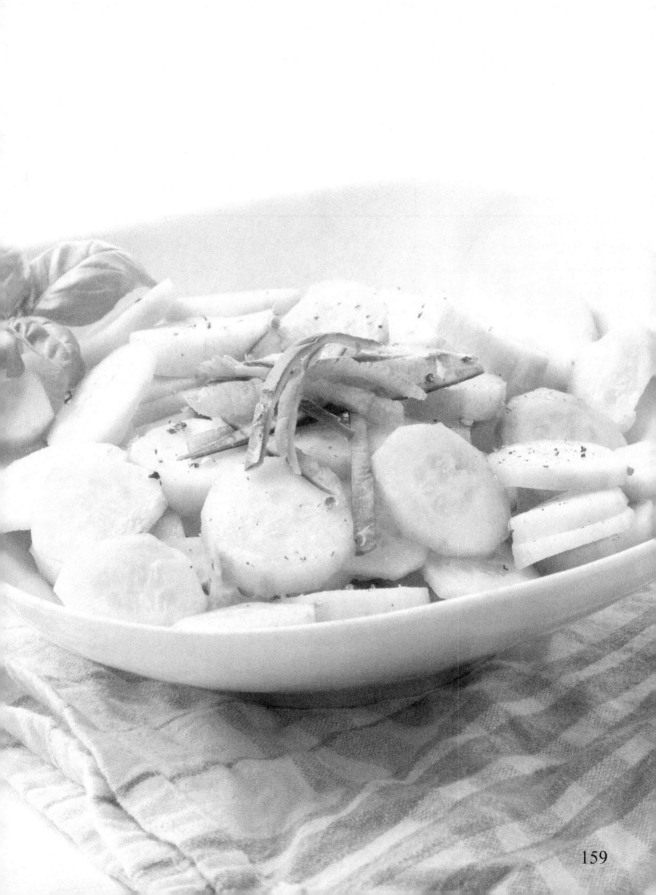

BAKED CARROT CHIPS

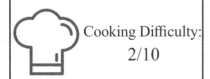 Cooking Difficulty: 2/10	Cooking Time: 15 minutes	Servings: 8

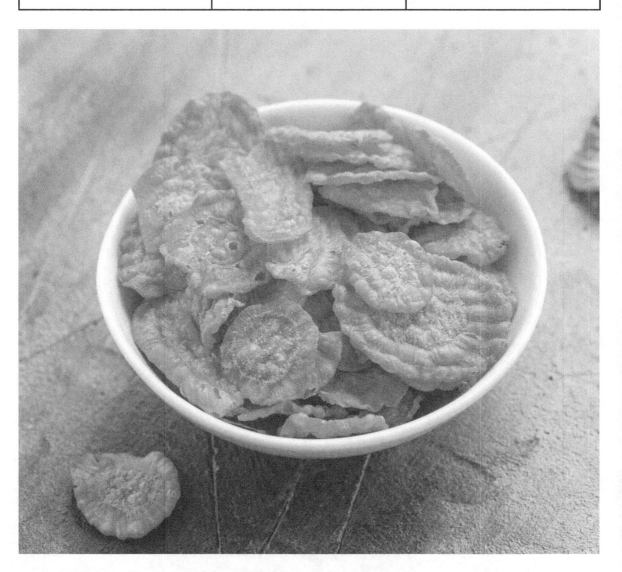

NUTRITIONAL INFORMATION
Calories: 100, Carbs: 12g, Fats: 8g, Proteins: 1g

INGREDIENTS

- ¼ c. olive oil
- 1 tsp. ground cinnamon
- 1 tsp. ground cumin
- salt
- 3 lbs. carrots

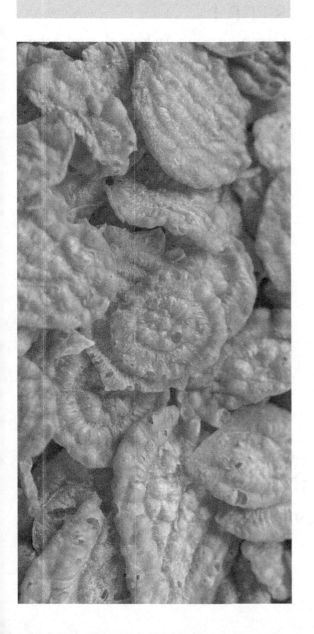

STEP 1

Heating your oven to 425 and setting up a baking sheet with some parchment paper.

STEP 2

Next, you will want to chop the top off each carrot and slice the carrot up paper-thin. You can complete this task by using a knife, but it typically is easier if you have a mandolin slicer.

STEP 3

Toss them in a small bowl with the cinnamon, cumin, olive oil, and a touch of salt. When the carrot slices are well coated, go ahead and lay them across your baking sheet.

STEP 4

Finally, pop the carrots into the oven for fifteen minutes. After this time, you may notice that the edges are going to start to curl and get crispy. At this point, remove the dish from the oven and flip all of the chips over. Return the dish into the oven for six or seven minutes, and then your chips will be set!

PEANUT BUTTER POPCORN

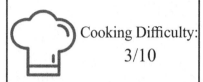 Cooking Difficulty: 3/10	Cooking Time: 12 minutes	Servings: 4

INGREDIENTS

- 2 tbsps. peanut oil
- ½ c. popcorn kernels
- ½ tsp. sea salt
- ⅓ c. peanut butter
- ¼ c. agave syrup
- ¼ c. honey

STEP 1
Combine popcorn kernels and peanut oil in a pot.

STEP 2
Over medium heat, shake the pot gently until all corn is popped.

STEP 3
In a saucepan, combine the honey and agave syrup. Cook over low heat for 5 min, then add the peanut butter and stir.

STEP 4
Coat the popcorn with prepared sauce.

NUTRITIONAL INFORMATION
430 Calories, 9g Protein, 20g Fat, 56g Carbs

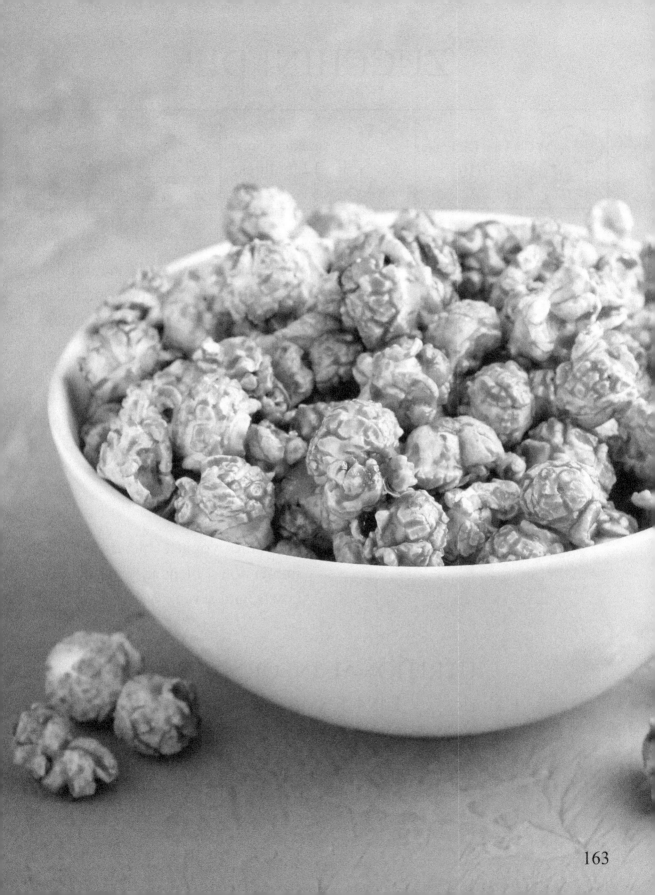

ZUCCHINI DIP

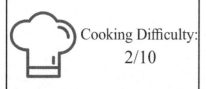 Cooking Difficulty: 2/10	Cooking Time: 12 minutes	Servings: 4

INGREDIENTS

- 2 spring onions, chopped
- ¼ c. veggie stock
- ¼ tsp. nutmeg, ground
- 2 garlic cloves, minced
- 2 zucchinis, chopped
- 1 tbsp. olive oil
- ½ c. yogurt, nonfat
- 1 tbsp. dill, chopped

STEP 1

Heat up a pan with the oil over medium heat, add the onions and garlic, stir and sauté for 3 minutes.

STEP 2

Add the zucchinis and the other ingredients except the yogurt, toss, cook for 7 minutes more and take off the heat.

STEP 3

Add the yogurt, blend using an immersion blender, divide into bowls, and serve.

NUTRITIONAL INFORMATION

Calories 76, Fat 4.1, Carbs 7.2, Protein 3.4

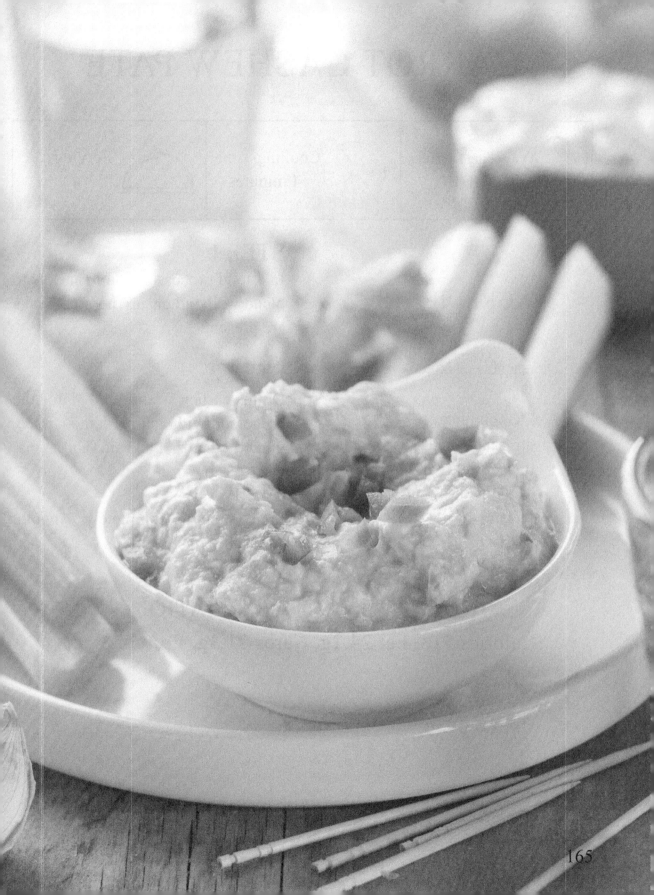

CARROT CASHEW PATE

 Cooking Difficulty: 1/10	 Cooking Time: 4 minutes	Servings: 4

INGREDIENTS

- 2 c. carrots, chopped
- 1 c. cashews, soaked
- ¼ c. tahini
- ¼ c. lemon juice
- 1 tbsp. peeled and grated ginger
- ½ cilantro stems and leaves
- ½ tsp. salt

STEP 1

In a food processor, add in carrots to blend well and ensure no big chunks are present.

STEP 2

Drain cashews and add into the processor with tahini, lemon juice, ginger, cilantro, and salt.

STEP 3

Process until completely smooth. Add salt to taste. Serve.

NUTRITIONAL INFORMATION

Calories 318, Fat 24.2g, Carbs 21.3g, Protein 8.6g

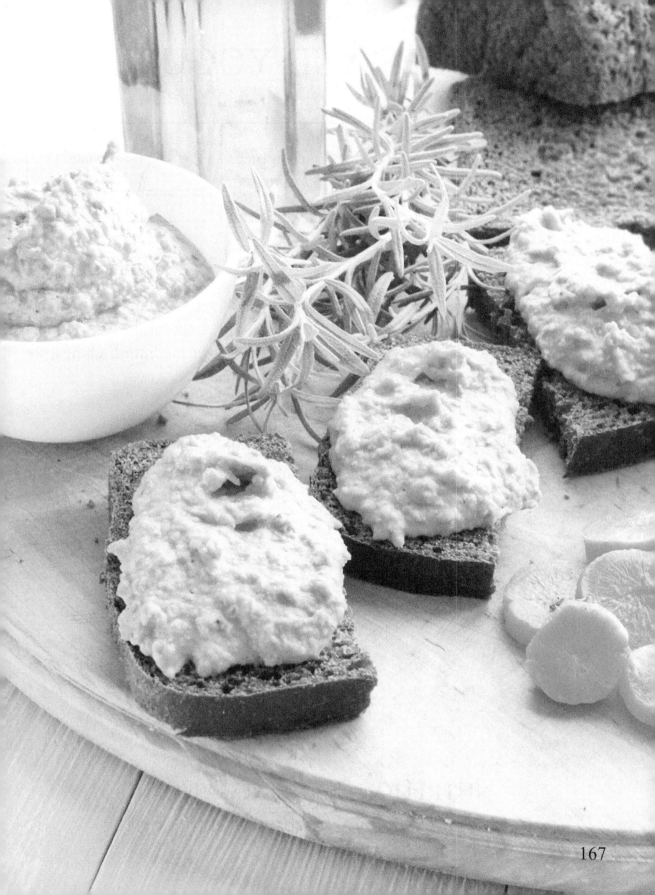

APPLES AND YOGURT

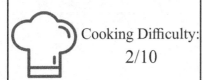 Cooking Difficulty: 2/10	Cooking Time: 37 minutes	Servings: 4

INGREDIENTS

- 1 c. yogurt
- 2 apples, cored, peeled and chopped
- 1 ½ c. oat milk
- 1 c. oats, steel cut
- ¼ c. maple syrup

STEP 1

In a pot, combine the oats with the milk and the other ingredients except the yogurt, toss, bring to a simmer and cook over medium-high heat for 15 minutes.

STEP 2

Divide the yogurt into bowls, divide the apples and oats mix on top and serve.

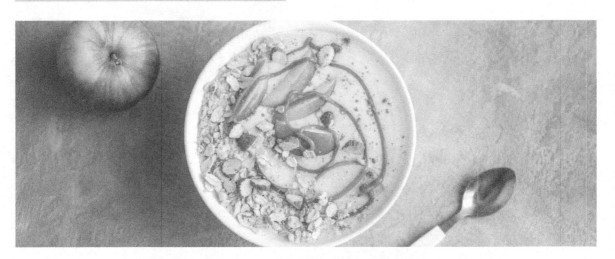

NUTRITIONAL INFORMATION

Calories 32, Fat 0.7g, Carbs 6.1g, Protein 1.1g

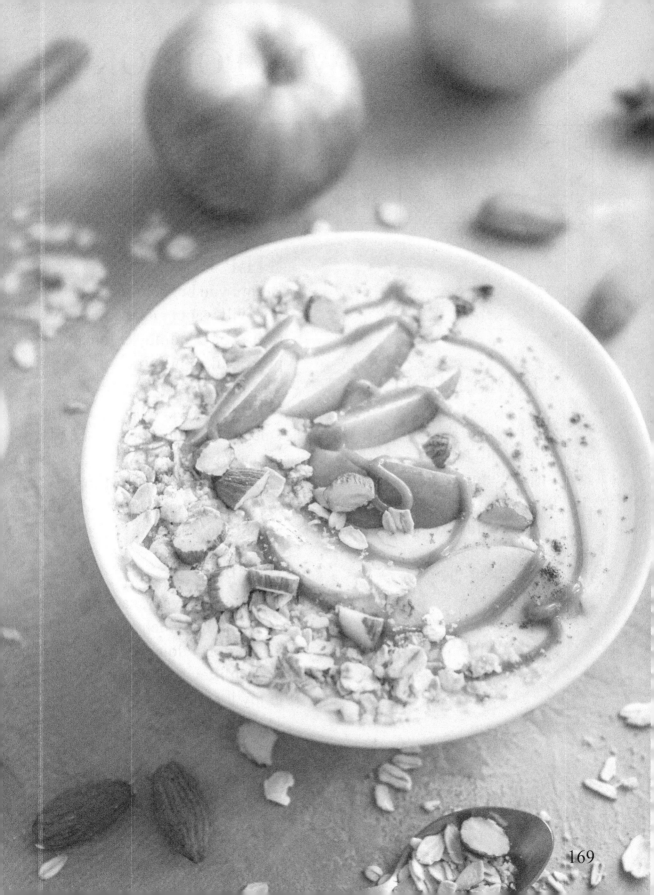

CAULIFLOWER POPCORN

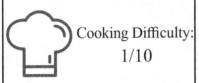 Cooking Difficulty: 1/10	Cooking Time: 480 minutes	Servings: 4

INGREDIENTS

- 2 tbsps. olive oil
- 2 tsps. chili powder
- 2 tsps. cumin
- 1 tbsp. nutritional yeast
- 1 head cauliflower
- salt

STEP 1

Before you begin making this recipe, you will want to take a few moments to cut your cauliflower into bite-sized pieces, like popcorn.

STEP 2

Once your cauliflower is set, place it into a mixing bowl and coat with the olive oil. Once coated properly, add in the nutritional yeast, salt, and the rest of the spices.

STEP 3

You can enjoy your snack immediately or place into a dehydrator at 115 for 8 hours. By doing this, it will make the cauliflower crispy! You can really enjoy it either way.

NUTRITIONAL INFORMATION
Calories: 100, Carbs: 10g, Fats: 5g, Proteins: 5g

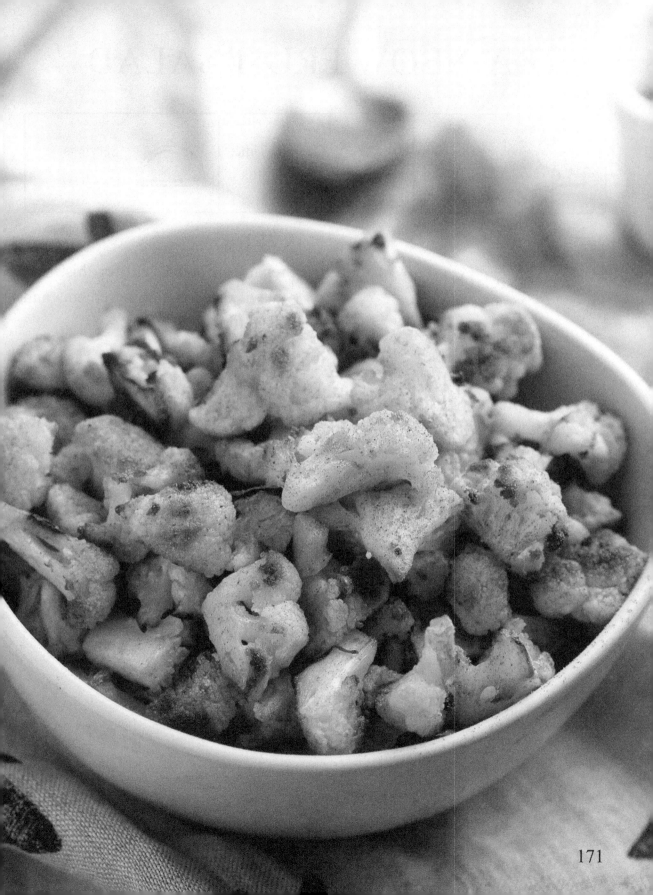

RAINBOW FRUIT SALAD

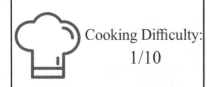 Cooking Difficulty: 1/10	Cooking Time: 5 minutes	Servings: 4

INGREDIENTS

for the fruit salad:
- 1 lb. hulled strawberries, sliced
- 1 c. kiwis, halved, cubed
- 1 ¼ c. blueberries
- 1 1/3 c. blackberries
- 1 c. pineapple chunks

for the maple lime dressing:
- 2 tsps. lime zest
- ¼ c. maple syrup
- 1 tbsp. lime juice

STEP 1
Prepare the salad, and for this, take a bowl, place all its ingredients and toss until mixed.

STEP 2
Prepare the dressing, and for this, take a small bowl, place all its ingredients and whisk well.

STEP 3
Drizzle the dressing over salad, toss until coated and serve.

NUTRITIONAL INFORMATION
Calories: 88.1, Fat: 0.4 g, Carbs: 22.6 g, Protein: 1.1 g

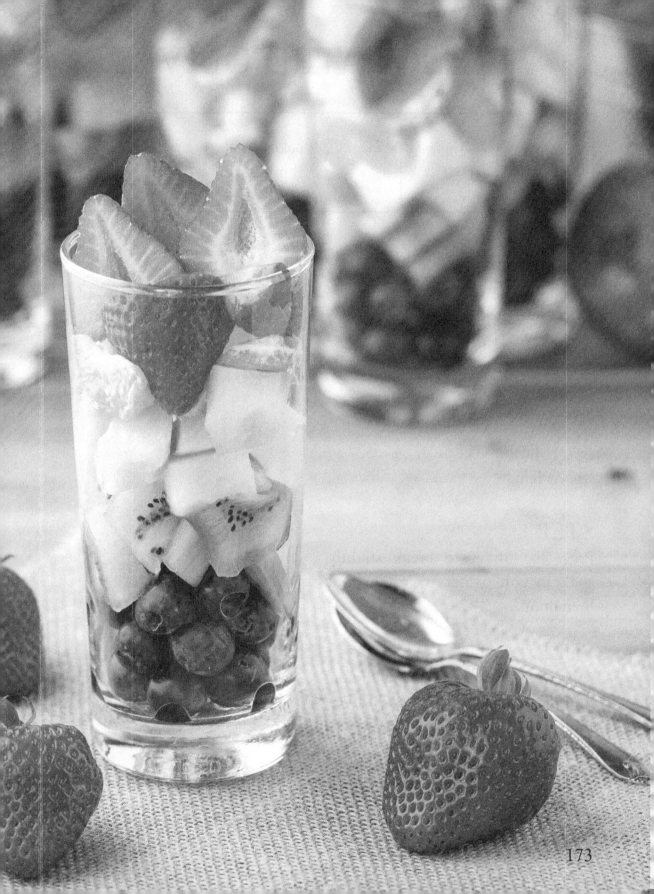

MARINATED OLIVES

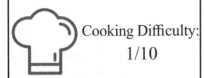 Cooking Difficulty: 1/10

 Cooking Time: 2 minutes

 Servings: 8

INGREDIENTS

- 1 1/3 c. green or tan olives
- 4 tbsps. chopped coriander
- 4 tbsps. chopped flat leaf parsley
- 1 crushed garlic clove
- 1 tsp. grated ginger
- 1 sliced red chili
- ¼ lemon

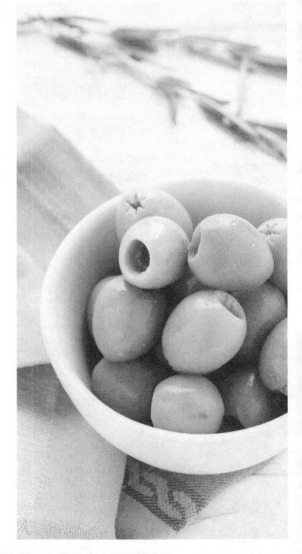

STEP 1

Press the olives to break slightly, soak in cold water overnight, and then drain.

STEP 2

Mix well the ingredients and pour into the jars to marinade the olives. Place the jar in the fridge for at least 1 week, shaking 2-3 time.

NUTRITIONAL INFORMATION

404.7 Calories, 40.0g Fats, 13.1g Net Carbs, 0.5g Protein

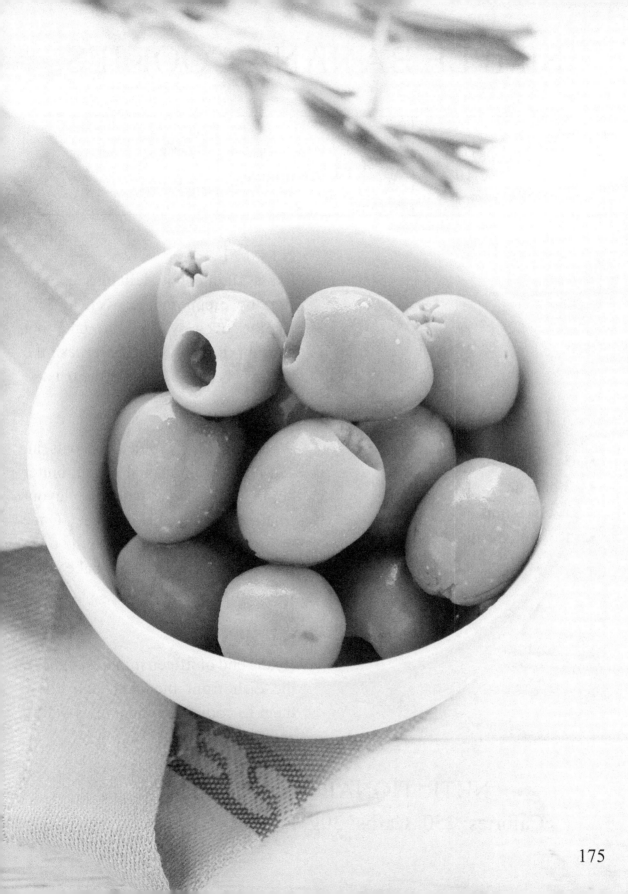

SIMPLE BANANA COOKIES

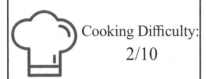 Cooking Difficulty: 2/10	Cooking Time: 16 minutes	Servings: 4

INGREDIENTS

- 3 tbsps. peanut butter
- 3 bananas
- ¼ c. walnuts
- 1 c. rolled oats

STEP 1

For a simple but delicious cookie, start by prepping the oven to 350. As the oven warms up, take out your mixing bowl and first mash the bananas before adding in the oats.

STEP 2

When you have folded the oats in, add in the walnuts and peanut butter before using your hands to layout small balls onto a baking sheet. Once this is set, pop the dish into the oven for fifteen minutes and bake your cookies.

STEP 3

By the end of fifteen minutes, remove the dish from the oven and allow them to cool for five minutes before enjoying.

NUTRITIONAL INFORMATION

Calories: 250, Carbs: 30g, Fats: 10g, Proteins: 5g

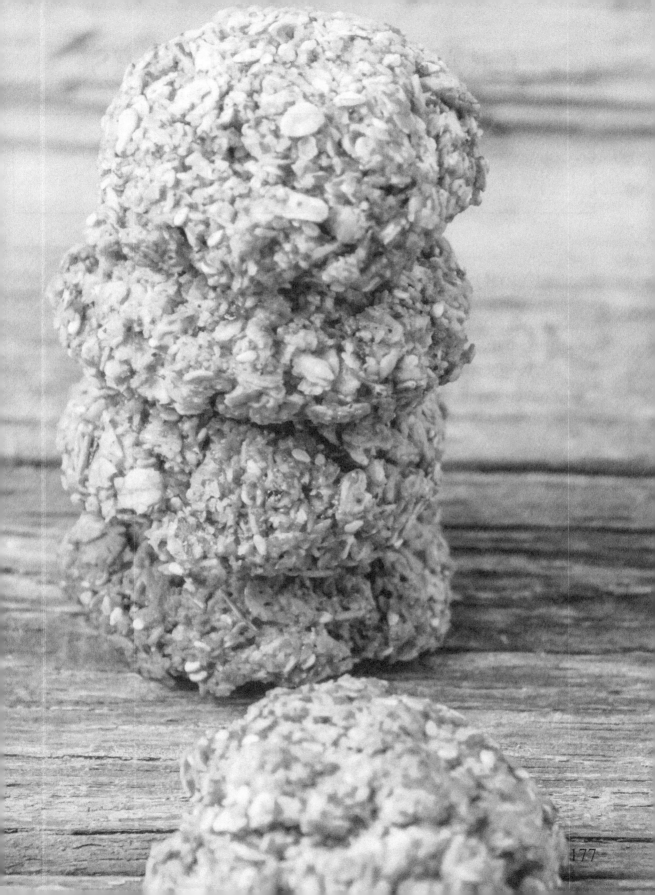

CRANBERRY SQUARES

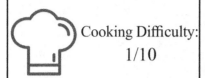 Cooking Difficulty: 1/10	Cooking Time: 4 minutes	Servings: 4

INGREDIENTS

- 2 tbsps. coconut, shredded
- 2 tbsps. rolled oats
- 1 c. cranberries
- 2 oz. coconut cream

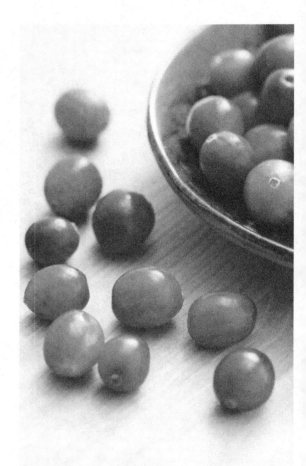

STEP 1

In a blender, combine the oats with the cranberries and the other ingredients, pulse well, and spread into a square pan.

STEP 2

Cut into squares and keep them in the fridge for 3 hours before serving.

NUTRITIONAL INFORMATION

Calories 32, Fat 0.7g, Carbs 6.1g, Protein 1.1g

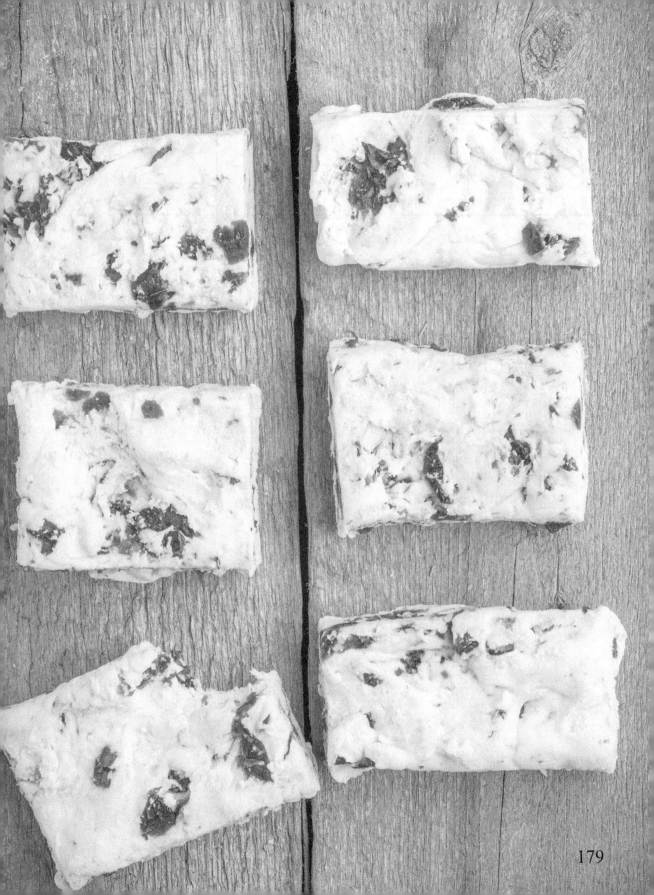

COOKIE DOUGH BITES

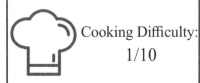 Cooking Difficulty: 1/10	Cooking Time: 5 minutes	Servings: 18

INGREDIENTS

- 15 oz. cooked chickpeas
- 1/3 c. vegan chocolate chips
- 1/3 c. and 2 tbsps. peanut butter
- 8 medjool dates pitted
- 1 tsp. vanilla extract, unsweetened
- 2 tbsps. maple syrup
- 1 ½ tbsps. almond milk, unsweetened

STEP 1

Place chickpeas in a food processor along with dates, butter, and vanilla and then process for 2 minutes until smooth.

STEP 2

Add remaining ingredients, except for chocolate chips, and then pulse for 1 minute until blends and dough comes together.

STEP 3

Add chocolate chips, stir until just mixed, then shape the mixture into 18 balls, optionally garnish with coconut flakes and refrigerate for 4 hours until firm. Serve straight away.

NUTRITIONAL INFORMATION

Calories: 200, Fat: 9 g, Carbs: 26 g, Protein: 1 g

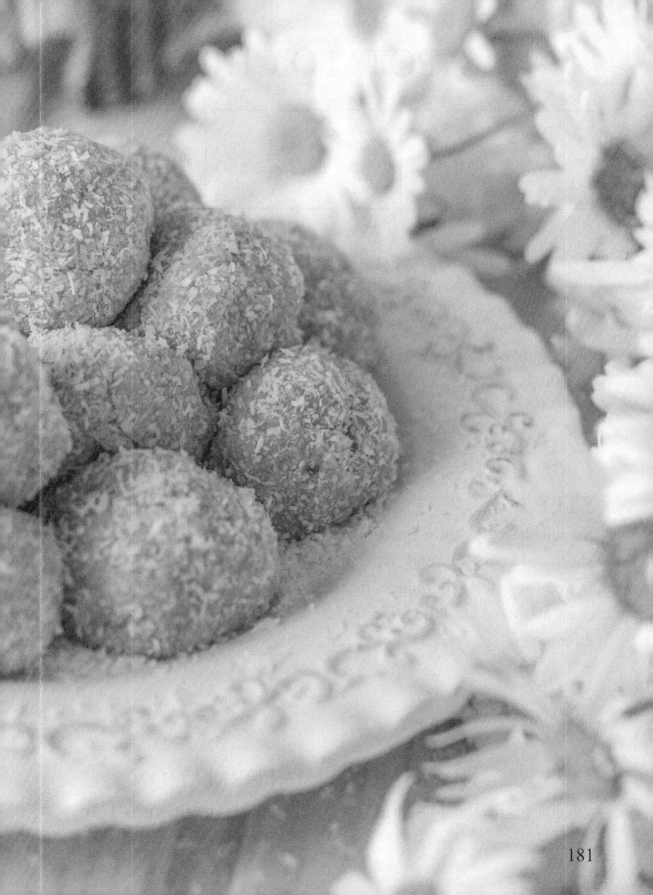

POTATO CHIPS

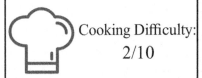 Cooking Difficulty: 2/10 Cooking Time: 21 minutes Servings: 4

INGREDIENTS

- 1 tsp. sweet paprika
- 1 tbsp. chives, chopped
- 4 gold potatoes, peeled and thinly sliced
- 2 tbsps. olive oil
- 1 tbsp. chili powder

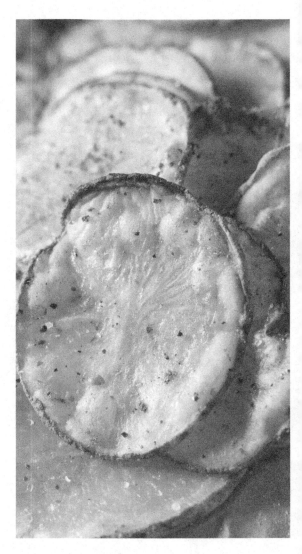

STEP 1

Spread the chips on a lined baking sheet, add the oil and the other ingredients, toss, introduce in the oven and bake at 390 degrees F for 20 minutes.

STEP 2

Divide into bowls and serve.

NUTRITIONAL INFORMATION
Calories 118, Fat 7.4g, Carbs 13.4g, Protein 1.3g

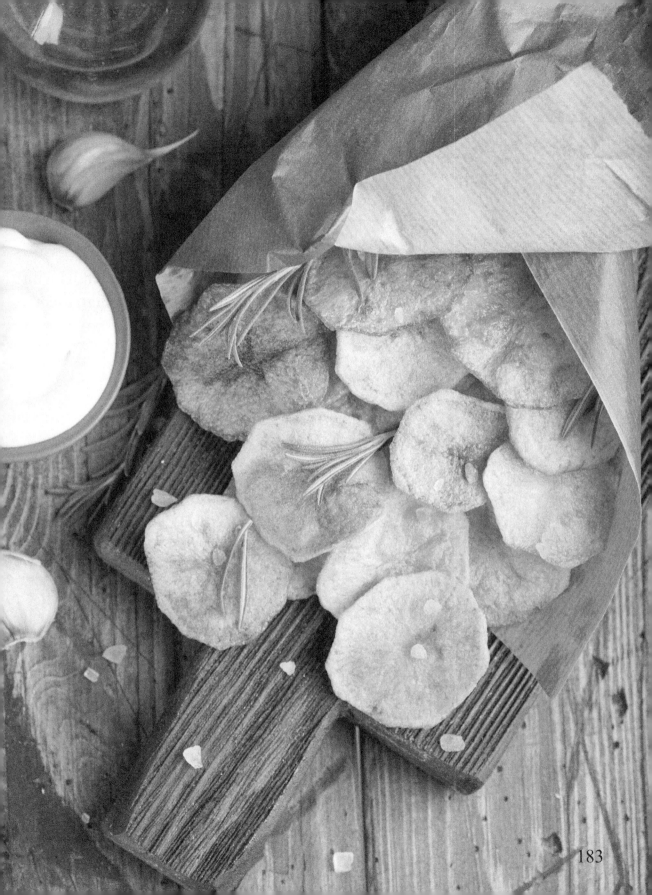

LENTILS SPREAD

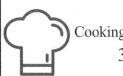 Cooking Difficulty: 3/10	Cooking Time: 15 minutes	Servings: 4

INGREDIENTS

- 2 garlic cloves, minced
- ½ c. cilantro, chopped
- 14 oz. canned lentils, drained, unsalted, and rinsed
- 1 lemon juice
- 2 tbsps. olive oil

STEP 1

In a blender, combine the lentils with the oil and the other ingredients, pulse well, divide into bowls and serve as a party spread.

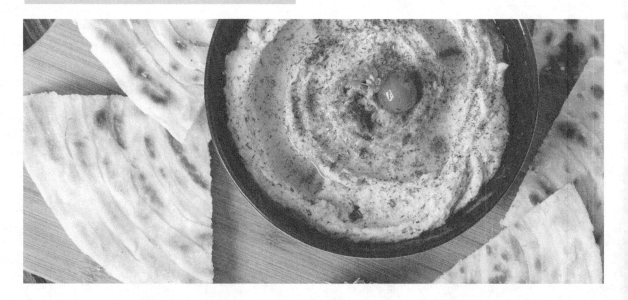

NUTRITIONAL INFORMATION

Calories 416, Fat 8.2g, Carbs 60.4g, Protein 25.8g

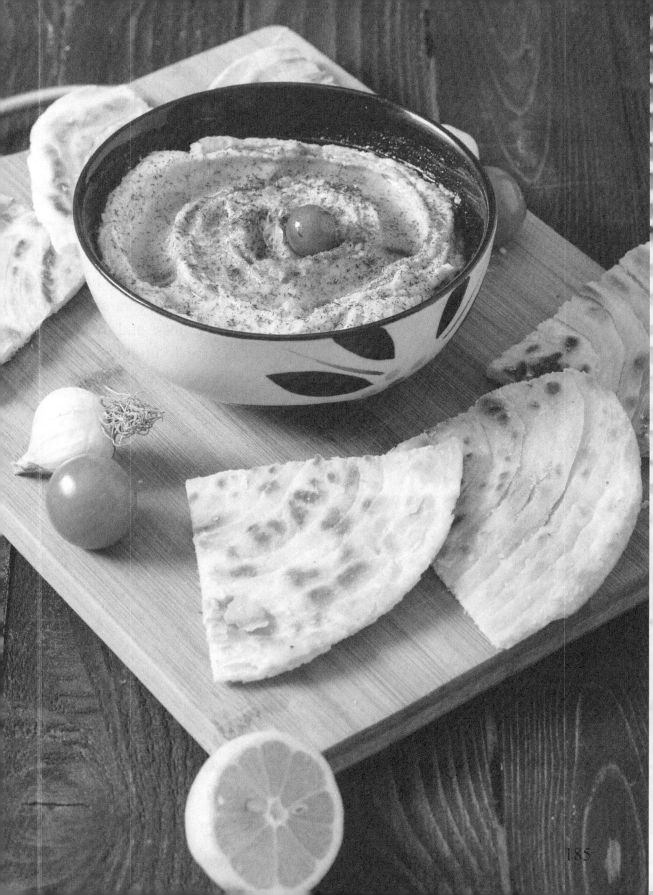

ROASTED WALNUTS

Cooking Difficulty: 1/10	Cooking Time: 15 minutes	Servings: 8

INGREDIENTS

- 14 oz. walnuts
- ½ tsp. garlic powder
- 1 tbsp. avocado oil
- ½ tsp. chili powder
- ½ tsp. smoked paprika
- ¼ tsp. cayenne pepper

STEP 1

Spread the walnuts on a lined baking sheet, add the paprika and the other ingredients, toss and bake at 410 degrees F for 15 minutes. Divide into bowls and serve as a snack.

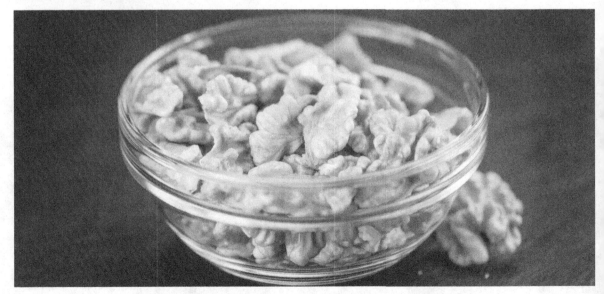

NUTRITIONAL INFORMATION
Calories 311, Fat 29.6g, Carbs 5.3g, Protein 12g

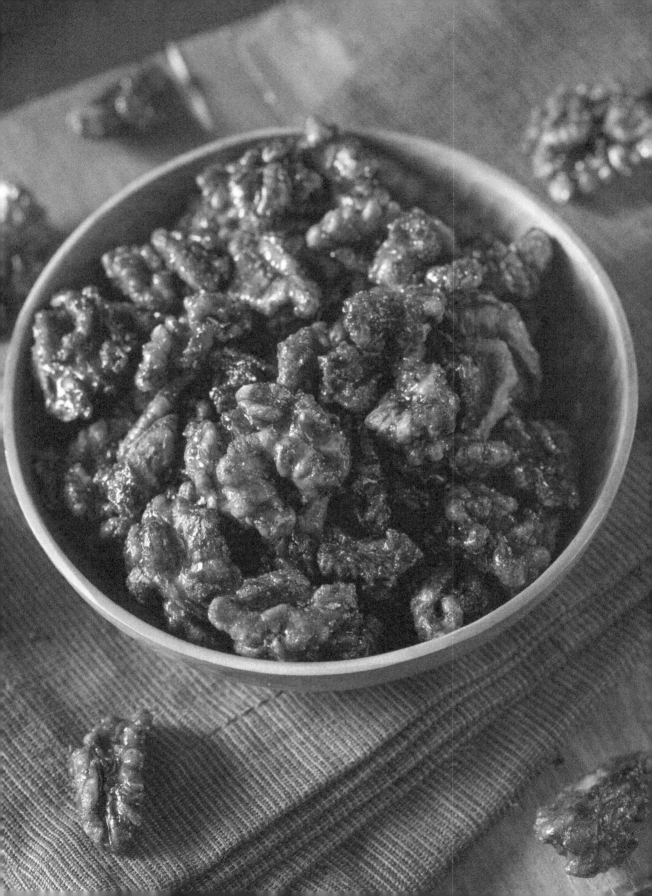

CONCLUSION

Every person is at risk of developing Alzheimer's disease and dementia. Some people who have a family history, are older than sixty-five, follow an unhealthy diet, have reduced physical activity, high cholesterol, and who smoke are at a higher risk.

It is never too early to start making good changes for your health. Following the MIND diet is the first step towards reducing the risk, but also providing your body and brain with healthy nutrients. Including fresh vegetables, fruits, nuts, olive oil, fish, and poultry in your weekly menu is the first step towards making the change.

Besides eating healthy nutrients, make sure that you start exercising regularly. Start with something as simple as a ten-minute walk around the block. You can make a mix of cardio and lifting; this way, you will maintain your weight and will keep your brain's health in good shape.

Your lifestyle should include things such as social interactions with your friends. We are all social creatures, and good social interactions are one of the ways to keep our brains happy and healthy.

Besides that, learn something new every day. The seven pillars I have mentioned in the chapters are crucial to help you stay healthy and lower the risk of this unwanted disease. Be sure to keep a balanced diet, sleep well, reduce stress, exercise, see your friends, maintain your vascular health, and stimulate yourself mentally.

I hope that this book helped you learn several important things that can help you keep your brain in good health and good shape. We are all exposed to the risk of developing it, but if you are dedicated to the seven pillars and the healthy MIND diet, you will benefit significantly.

In the end, I want to thank you for reading this book. Follow the diet, be active and social, reduce your stress levels, and make sure that you keep yourself busy by doing what you love, surrounded with the people who love you and make you happy.

Garry Goodman

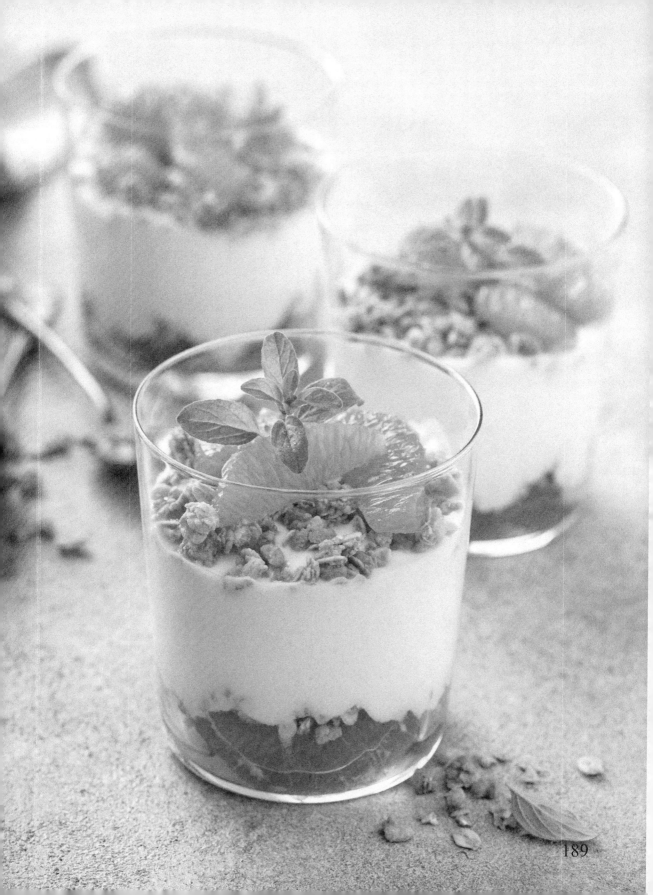

Made in the USA
Las Vegas, NV
07 January 2024

84025361R00105